754

MW00380816

C

Zero-Variable Theories and the Psychology of the Explainer

Robert A. Wicklund

Zero-Variable Theories and the Psychology of the Explainer

Springer-Verlag
New York Berlin Heidelberg
London Paris Tokyo Hong Kong

Robert A. Wicklund
Abteilung Psychologie
Universität Bielefeld
Federal Republic of Germany

Library of Congress Cataloging-in-Publication Data

Wicklund, Robert A.
    Zero-variable theories and the psychology of the explainer /
Robert A. Wicklund.
        p.   cm.
    1. Psychology—Philosophy.   2. Psychologists—Psychology.
3. Explanation.   I. Title.
BF38.W736   1990
150′.1—dc20   89-39733

Typeset by Asco Trade Typesetting, Hong Kong.
Printed and bound by Edwards Brothers, Ann Arbor, Michigan.
Printed in the United States of America.

9 8 7 6 5 4 3 2 1

ISBN 0-387-97165-3 Springer-Verlag New York Berlin Heidelberg
ISBN 3-540-97165-3 Springer-Verlag Berlin Heidelberg New York

Preface

The reader should not suppose that this is a book about the philosophy of social science, or about moral pronouncements on what is good and bad in ancient and current psychological theorizing. Instead, the reader is invited to consider the psychological side of the *explainer*. What brings individuals, whether they carry the label *scientist in psychology* or not, to neglect the psychological perspective of those who are being explained? What is responsible for the explainer reducing complex behavioral patterns to "The person is a demagogue type" or "All people from hot climates do that"? And still another question: Are such oversimplifications part of the explainer's attempt to bring a quick, indelible order to the universe of human behavior?

The opening chapter introduces the explainer as someone whose directions of explaining are affected by control threats, incompetencies, and lack of experience. Such threats and incompetencies bring the explainer to account for others' actions by simplifying the others, treating them as static entities, with the result that deciding factors in their psychological backgrounds are neglected.

Psychology has characteristically limited its explaining of the explainer to the "everyday explainer," that is, to the so-called naive scientist. But why not extend our understanding of the explainer to all of those who try to come to terms with complex behavior, including those who carry the label *scientist*? This book assumes, without reservation, that the principles used to understand "naive explainers" can be applied just as well to "professional" explainers. Its chapters follow the course of development of the modern theory, as promulgated by scientifically working psychologists, and devote special attention to the narrow thinking that is so evident in recent efforts to capture and explain complex human action. It is shown that modern, widely published explanations manifest a style of theorizing that carries the following characteristics:

1. The humans who are being explained are first placed into fixed categories.

2. The explainer implements a single, home-grown categorizing instrument for this purpose.
3. These categories consist of lists of behaviors that appear to belong together (e.g., "honest," "loyal," "consistent").
4. The behaviors of category members, thus respondents in research projects, are then explained fully by those respondents' membership in one or the other category.
5. The explainer defends the categories as one would defend a territory, misusing statistical devices to demonstrate that other explainers cannot account for the behaviors of category members.
6. This direction of theory development, referred to here as the *zero-variable* theory, neglects the perspective of the person whose behaviors are being accounted for and also hinders integration among psychological explanations.

These fourteen chapters attempt to understand this development in explaining/theorizing, using the broad concepts of the explainer's *commitment* to a fixed portrait of the human, the explainer's *control needs* with respect to complex human behavior, and the *competition* that stems from a field loaded with professional explainers. The final chapter addresses the cultural side of these progressive simplifications and downfalls in theorizing and explanation and comes to the conclusion that a competitive, highly technical society produces the directions that are now explicit in the modern zero-variable theory.

Acknowledgments

The kernel of much that is written here can be traced back to numerous discussions between the author and Peter M. Gollwitzer, most of these talks occurring between the years 1983 and 1987. Our brainstormings culminated in a critique and an exchange, published in 1987.

The present writings necessitated the author's trying to become familiar with a number of areas that traditionally belong to classical personality theory, and a debt of gratitude is owed to Alois Angleitner, whose wisdom in those areas often served as a corrective, and was always enlightening.

Wolf Nowack, Marion Scheuer, and Melvin L. Snyder not only expressed their interest in the development of the book as it proceeded, but they also read an entire first draft and were generous with opinions and constructive critiques. Discussions with Günter Bierbrauer proved to be informative for certain theoretical aspects of the manuscript; his input is gratefully acknowledged.

The central figure in the production of this book was Mrs. Katharina Schaadt. Her typing and editing skills have been exemplary; her spirit has been motivating.

Robert A. Wicklund

Contents

1
An Introduction to the Psychology of the Explainer

The *explainer*, the central topic of this and the following chapters, is not necessarily the person who creates a hierarchical explanatory system, out of interwoven concepts drawn from different levels of abstraction, in the manner of idealized theory; the explainer here is the observer of behavior, particularly complex human behavior, and is defined through the simple act of characterizing others' behaviors and behavioral tendencies. It is not important whether we apply the term *explain*, *sort out*, *define* or *characterize*. For the present, the central figure is the everyday observer of the human who then comments, in more or less sophisticated style, on that which is observed. What is "more or less sophisticated"? For a start, let's try out two cases of observer acounts for observed behavior.

Case A (The Simple)

Staying at a very concrete, visible level, the explainer notes the shape and form of the other's behavior, as well as the shape and form of the *person* who has behaved. For example, the target person (a politician) who is party to a debate is observed to interrupt the opponent, not allowing the opponent to finish a single sentence. The person is then characterized, for example, "This is a highly aggressive politician," or "This is a highly argumentative type." Or, if the target person exhibits obvious external characteristics, the observation might read, "Typical for people of that race, of that age, of that nationality."

Although psychologists would be prone to regard such forms of explanation as incomplete, childish, or at best "implicit" (see Wegner & Vallacher, 1977), these approaches to explanation, albeit in slightly cloaked form, are remarkably common within the psychology of complex human behavior. A behavior or set of behaviors is observed within a given realm and some fixed, highly visible aspect of the person is then given as the adequate characterization.

Case B (More Complex and Behind the Scenes)

In explaining the politician's seemingly obtrusive debating style, the explainer in Case B makes recourse to the politician's background. This simple distinction—reference to the background or not—is the kernel of the difference between Cases A and B. But the distinction can be drawn still further. Looking behind the scenes of the behavior is not limited to empirical facts lying within the target person's background; it can also mean considering the *psychological condition* of the person.[1] The term *psychological condition* means the politician's perceptions, memory contents, motivations, wishes, conflicts, and the like. Thus, rather than limiting one's explanation to concrete, visible aspects of the target person, the explainer in Case B refers to the inner mental life (e.g., perceptions and motivations) of the person being observed.[2]

Perspective Taking

The difference between Cases A and B is, perhaps more simply stated, a difference in the extent of taking or imagining the other's perspective. If we think for a moment about the components the target person (the politician) brings to the debate situation, no reasonable psychologist or other person would deny the following list: one's ordinary biographical history, particular motives (to win, to make a favorable impression, to get the debate over with), perceptions of the debate opponent, habitual styles of perceiving one's opponent, a certain verbal repertoire, and interaction style, all implanted relatively early, plus innumerable other components of the person. The Case A explanation neglects *all* of these aspects by characterizing the behavior in terms of the speaker's race, nationality, or in terms of a trait ("aggressive") that simply renames the behavior enacted. The Case A explanation disregards prior happenings in the individual's past; more important, it shunts aside the manifold facets of the politician's psychological condition. These background facets (earlier debate encounters, motivations, perceptions) are the politician's *perspective*. The more complex form of explanation (Case B) considers such perspectives; thus, we might say tentatively that perspective-taking readiness is roughly on the same level as the readiness to offer more psychological explanations of another's behavior.

In speaking of the psychologist's task as one of taking a perspective, it would not be correct to say that this perspective could be reported by the respondents who are being studied. No doubt all people, as self-observers, can report quite extensively on their backgrounds, motivations, and perceptions, but the goal of the psychologist is not to produce an explanation that coincides exactly with the *subject's* or *patient's* self-descriptions.

The reasons should be apparent: the self-observer (e.g., the research respondent) cannot form the criteria for judging whether scientific statements about human behavior are correct; psychological laws must ultimately come to terms with the mental processes and behavior of young children (who are quite limited in their self-reports), and with mental processes, behaviors, and background factors that are not necessarily part of each person's self-knowledge. That people err, and often quite radically, in reporting features of their backgrounds, their mental states, and their behavioral dispositions, is common knowledge in the psychological literature (Fazio & Zanna, 1978; Fischhoff, 1982; Fiske & Taylor, 1984; Gibbons, 1990; Nisbett & Wilson, 1977).

This line of thought has a simple implication: in speaking of the psychologist's task as one of comprehending the perspective of the respondent, *perspective* should not be equated with what respondents say about themselves. Rather, the perspective of the respondent—for a scientific psychology—consists of the multitude of past experiences, conflicts, perceptions, motivations, and other events that govern the thinking and behavior of the individual. It is the psychologist's task to gain insight into the course of these events, whereby the respondent's self-report about such processes is little more than a starting point into understanding such processes.

If psychological explanations entail the explainer's looking behind the overt appearance of the target person and into the multifaceted aspects of the individual's psychological condition, it stands to reason that we could discuss the *explainer's* psychological aspects. That is, the tendency of people, as explainers, to implement (1) a simplified mode of explanation or, alternatively, (2) a behind-the-scenes, perspective-taking mode of explanation, should be seen in itself as a psychological problem. To be sure, several theoretical directions have a good deal to say about the explainer's readiness or capabilities in taking the other's perspective, and thus the readiness to move toward the Case B form of explanation of behavior.

Promoting Perspective Taking: Age, Culture, and Induction of Empathy

It is no secret that the naked biological factor of age is related to children's capacity to consider the other's perspective. Thus in examples from Piaget (1924) and Piaget and Inhelder (1956), children show rapid increments in readiness to grasp the sense of another's geographical position, relative to their own positions. A child at a relatively early age who stands on one side of a toy mountain is inclined to assume that others (standing on the opposite side of the mountain) can view exactly the same scene. After the age of about eight years (and here there is considerable debate about age factors) the child is more ready to realize that others do not always view his own perspective (Coie, Costanzo, & Franhill, 1973; Feffer, 1959; Mossler, Marvin, & Greenberg, 1976).

Age in and of itself can hardly be considered as a psychological contributor to perspective-taking capacity; normally one talks about "cognitive development," assuming that the child's cognitive capacities gradually ripen, eventually reaching the point at which one's own perspective is separated from those of others, thus ending the egocentric fusion between the two.

A more concrete formulation is found in a fascinating field study by Hollos and Cowan (1973). Norwegian children of different ages were studied in three kinds of locations: one in a small city, the second a village with about 1400 people, and the third an isolated mountain community (Slettås), in which the possibility of contact with other children was minimal. In the words of Hollos and Cowan, most of the families in the Slettås area lived far from one another, precluding frequent contact between families. The children were characterized as spending most of their time alone or observing others and, interestingly, also showed minimal verbal contact with one another.

All of the children were tested for perspective-taking ability by means of several tests, one of which is a well-known invention of Flavell (1968). First, the child views a meaningful series of seven pictures, which together constitute a clear story line. The child then tells a story based on the seven pictures. Subsequently three of the pictures are removed, thereby altering the nature of the story. Then another person enters the room, sees the new (shortened) series of pictures, and the child is asked to tell the story in the same manner as this person would tell it. The study showed marked differences between Slettås children and village or city children: the frequency of regular social contact bore a direct relation to the ability or readiness to acknowledge that the second person had seen only four of the seven pictures. The children who lacked early experience and contact with others were inclined simply to project their own interpretations, rather than considering the context (i.e., that the other person had seen three pictures fewer).

This Norwegian observation has direct relevance for our primary theme—the *explainer*. Socially impoverished children are simply very poor psychologists, in the sense of not being able to infer what another person perceives. Placed in the position of having to ascertain another's thoughts, they are relatively incapable of drawing on pertinent characteristics of the environment that would certainly influence the other's thoughts. The alternative, of course, is simply to assume the other would think the same thoughts as themselves. The more urban groups of children, in contrast, were in the position to draw on critical features of the context to infer what the other had perceived and learned, and thus the story that person would relate.[3]

The study implies that the depth of the explainer's observations can be improved by moving the explainer's (child's) cognitions in the direction of others' standpoints. "Contact," per se, does not mean very much psychologically, but one critical aspect of interpersonal contact may be that one devotes more time to thinking about others' plights, situations, or psychological states. The research on empathy induction takes this focus idea quite literally; subjects are verbally instructed to think about the plight, background conditions, or emotions of the other (see a summary by Wispé, 1986). To be sure, such instructions do have an impact on helping behavior, mediated through one's cognizance of the other's psychological states (Batson 1987).

Highly pertinent here is a study by Storms (1973), in which the subject's task was to analyze the behavior of a target person. If the subject's attention was on the face of the target person, the subject tended to account for the behavior in terms of broad dispositions. However, if the subject's attention was on the *interaction partner* of the target person, the explanation shifted in the direction of a contextual one, that is, the explanation took into account the target person's social context. Interestingly, the explanations in this latter condition were also more in line with target persons' own explanations for their own behavior.

If we piece these three elements together—the Norwegian children, the empathy induction, and the experiment by Storms—we begin to see a potential connection between the explainer's own background and the kinds of explanations that are offered for others' behavior. A context that promotes the explainer's "taking part" in the target person's situation also promotes the perspective-taking response in that (1) the explanation then corresponds more to actual factors within the other's background and (2) the explanation comes to acknowledge the target person's *own* account of what is going on, as opposed to reducing the target person to a simple, static role (e.g., always aggressive). To the extent that the explainer's nose is not pushed toward the target person's situation, the explanation disregards the special character of the other's background and attends more to stable aspects of the target person, as in the Storms study. But this is only a start; still further considerations exist regarding the psychological background of the explainer who refers to the other's perspective.

Self-Focused Attention

It was Piaget's (1924) observation that the egocentric, non-perspective-taking orientation of young children has to do with a lack of the facility to grasp the uniqueness of one's own perspective or self. Theoretically, the onset of perspective-taking skills is signaled by the break-up of two previously fused elements—one's own distinct viewpoint and alternative viewpoints. While such increments in self-focus are supposed to accompany the child's natural development, one can also regard the self-focus variable as a dimension that remains active into adulthood. For instance, if adults are brought to train their visual or auditory attention on their own selves, there are definite increments in perspective-taking performance, whether measured by means of the Norway study techniques (originally taken from Flavell, 1968) or other methods. Altogether, seven such experiments are reported by Hass (1984) and Stephenson and Wicklund (1983, 1984).

A simple example of this process stems from the second experiment reported by Hass (1984), who used a paradigm resembling the left/right perspective-taking tasks first suggested by Piaget (1924). Piaget's version of the paradigm involved the experimenter's asking the child to "show me my right hand. Now my left. Show me my right leg, now my left." (p. 98). Piaget found that most of his youthful subjects were capable of handling these perspective-taking tasks by the age of eight years. The Hass (1984) counterpart to Piaget required subjects to draw the letter "E" on their foreheads. The perspective-taking measure was simply the proportion of subjects who drew the "E" in a nonegocentric matter, thus for another's perspective. Even though the participants were well over eight years of age, only 17 percent of them drew the "E" so that a person hypothetically facing the subject would be able to read it. However, when self-awareness was induced by means of a TV camera (positioned behind the subject's head), 48 percent of the student-subjects drew the "E" for the hypothetical other's perspective.

Why should self-focused attention contribute positively to perspective-taking performance? It sounds almost paradoxical, in that we have already suggested that directing attention toward the *other's situation* promotes perspective taking. Theoretically, it works as follows: To analyze another person without being influenced by the constituents of one's own self, it is necessary that one's own self be differentiated from others. Since this differentiation is not necessarily achieved once and for all after the "magic" Piagian age of six years or so (see Piaget & Inhelder, 1956), it becomes necessary to reinstitute provocations to self-awareness, to ensure that the individuals not simply fuse their own manner of thinking or perceiving with estimates about what others think.

Therefore, to create a maximal and nonegocentric orientation toward another's perspective, we need two kinds of elements. One element is knowledge of the other's context or background, which in part is a question of contact with others and a cognitive orientation toward their contexts (the Norway study; Storms, 1973). Second, the tendency to oversimplify one's perceptions of another by way of egocentrism can be reduced through an increment in self-focus. The result should be increased differentiation between one's own mental states or background and observations about the mental states and backgrounds of others.

Factors that Intrude on the Perspective-Taking Facilities of the Explainer

The preceding discussion is the more optimistic side of this first chapter; thus far we have assumed that, if the social conditions are right, individuals will blossom into explainers who look beyond their own views and can extrapolate to the other's background, searching out bases for inferring or deriving the other's motives, perceptions, habits, and other psychological components. But there are also destructive factors, interfering with the explainer's progress as we have thus far idealized it, factors that are quite well grounded in theory and in empirical work. What do they look like?

General Threats to the Ego

The psychological background of the Adorno, Frenkel-Brunswick, Levinson, and Sanford (1950) work on the authoritarian personality brings us to certain socially based factors that appear to underlie the person's tendencies along our Case A (simplicity) to Case B (complex) dimension. The starting point for Adorno and colleagues (1950) was the assumption that parents who suffer under the threat of status-anxiety are inclined to adopt particular world views that (1) are discriminatory regarding outgroups (2) and reflect a rigidity in the analysis of human behavior (see Brown, 1965). The famous "fascism" scale of Adorno et al. includes items that have much to do with the style of the explainer. For instance, "Some people are born with an urge to jump from high places"; "People can be divided into two distinct classes: the weak and the strong"; "Some day it will probably be shown that astrology can explain a lot of things"; "Most people don't realize how much our lives are controlled by plots hatched in secret places" (Robinson & Shaver, 1969, p. 316). The person who assents to such items, according to the theory of Adorno et al., suffers from status anxiety and threats to a sense of self-worth. Thus, the starting point is a kind of ego-threat, based in this case on status relations, and is reflected in a rigid view of others. The authoritarian person, as defined in the contexts of the Adorno scales, is against introspection or analysis of psychological states and favors a view of the human that represents a non-changing, permanent essence—an essence that is transmitted via such visible entities as generations and race. Individuality, in the sense of a person's single motives, habits, perceptions, and personality traits, is neglected and supplanted through broad, socially defined categories (race, gender, age, religious persuasion). In short, the work of Adorno et al. implies that the status-threatened individual comes to "explain" others in terms of a simplified method, similar to our Case A, neglecting the background and psychological condition of the person being addressed.

A most informative derivation from the Adorno et al. thinking was brought to light in a study by Steiner (1954). Subjects were confronted with pairs of person descriptors, some of which did not, at first glance, seem to fit together. Steiner assessed the extent to which subjects allowed that each pair of traits could occur within the same unit, and found, quite convincingly, that the more authoritarian subjects of his sample rejected trait pairs that were internally inconsistent.

This kind of thinking is given more explicit theoretical treatment in the work of Easterbrook (1959), who addressed the issue of "the effects of emotion on cue utilization." The general idea resembles a generalization of the status-threat notion of Adorno et al.: The starting point is a strong emotional state, a conflict, an ego-threat, or similar imposition on one's cognitive functioning. The outcome is a narrowing of the perceptual field. This means that a potential explainer who is emotionally upset, in a state of conflict, whose control is threatened, or is frustrated, tends toward a simplified explanation of others' behavior—one that would disregard complex factors, particularly hidden or background factors. In short, the elements pertinent to the total perspective of the person being analyzed would be disregarded.

Threat to Control and Mode of Explaining: Evidence for the Easterbrook Thesis

The number of experiments in psychology that have assessed different modes of "explaining-behavior" is minimal, and the primary dimension on which these experiments have focused has been called "situational versus dispositional." Thus, "the boy was polite in the store because he had been instructed carefully in such matters by his parents" or "the boy was polite because he is a well-mannered, friendly child." "She shouted at the other driver because she was provoked," or "she shouted at the other driver because she is an aggressive sort." Sometimes the form of measurement is simplified, in that the respondent must indicate when the behavior generally depends on external factors or on the actor's permanent dispositions. In other cases the primary measure is simply the number or extent of dispositions that are named or checked off.

The important issue in the context of the *explainer* is, of course, what does the situation-versus-disposition dimension have to do with the perspective-taking issue just discussed? In part, the answer is easy to come by: (1) If the explainer has access to aspects of the individual's situation that are pertinent to the behavior and then neglects them, the neglect of the pertinent perspective is apparent. This is the essence of the paradigm we saw in the context of the Norwegian study. (2) If the *dispositional* explanation for behavior is nothing more than a summary statement of behavior ("The woman shouted at the other driver; the reason is her aggressiveness."), then the perspective has been totally neglected. In other words, a summing up of the behavioral instance in terms of person descriptors such as "aggressive," "crude," and "emotional" is in no manner based on the background of the target person.

In experiments by Berscheid, Graziano, Monson, and Dermer (1976), Miller and Norman (1975), and Miller, Norman, and Wright (1978), the subject was treated as an explainer. The idea in the Berscheid et al. study was for the subject to observe a specific other person, within the context of a discussion, and then give accounts for that person's discussion-behavior, particularly in terms of traits (e.g., "strong–weak"). The central beginning point for the research was threat-to-control; here we pick up the Adorno et al. (1950) and Easterbrook (1959) theme once again. The threat to control was defined through subjects' knowledge that they would later have a date with a given target person. It suffices to say that they should have felt a certain apprehension, thus threat to control, at the prospect of interacting with an unknown person.

Given that a date with the target person was expected, subjects' explanations for the target person's prior discussion-behavior resided more in dispositional terms ("strong" and the like); the trait ratings were significantly more extreme. Thus, the subjects ascribed a permanent essence to the target person without any objective basis. The authors' interpretation of this line of research was quite straightforward: An observer who expects further interaction with the observed person is threatened, and thus tries to regain a sense of control by rendering the other person stable. The more the other can be transformed into a stable, unwavering entity, the fewer surprises the observer would have in interacting with that person.

Ascribing a stable essence to someone is viewed by Berscheid et al. (1976) and also by Miller and colleagues (1975, 1978) as the active effort to exert control over an uncertain encounter with another person. This point is graphically underlined in a study by Miller et al. (1978), in which the extent of expected interaction was again varied. Control threat resulted in an increase in subjects' thinking that the future behavior of the target would be predictable, an effect that was particularly strong among subjects with a high chronic need for control (Rotter, 1966).

Also close to the thesis that control needs, ego-involvements, or conflicts can reduce one's sensitivity as an explainer is a study by Vallacher (1977). The respondents were asked to make ratings of a job interviewee, and during the course of making these judgments some of the subjects were observed themselves, with TV cameras trained on them. Vallacher reports marked differences in the way these two groups analyzed their target persons. The nonobserved subjects used many intervals along the *competence* dimension, discriminating effectively among the interviewees. In contrast, the observed subjects tended more to make either/or judgments. It is suggested that "the awareness of being observed can reduce the amount of information we attend to in someone . . ." (Wegner & Vallacher, 1977,

p. 86). The connection to Easterbrook's (1959) broad thesis is evident—an emotional state results in a kind of tunnel vision.

Thus the explainer, given the task of sorting out causal factors behind another's behavior, tends to move toward simplicity when confronted with threats to control. The observed behavior is summed up in adjectives that are assumed to apply indefinitely to the target person.

A parallel finding is noted by Funder (1980). Funder's primary interest was in the personality traits of the person who explains. The central question of his investigation was, "Does a person's personality determine whether he tends to explain more in terms of situations or in terms of chronic dispositions?" Based on ratings from subjects' acquaintances, Funder was able to obtain personality data on his subjects regarding such qualities as "feels a lack of personal meaning in life," "thin-skinned," "sensitive to criticism," "does not cope well under stress," "basically anxious," "self-defensive," "lacks sense of humor," and others. If we regard such qualities through the perspective of Easterbrook (1959), we arrive at a very simple deduction: the thin-skinned, conflict-ridden, anxious, socially inept person who attempts to explain others' behavior should approach the task of explanation with tunnel vision. That is, rather than being attuned to what the target persons themselves perceive, thus to various contextual features, there should be a tendency to simplify. And if the research of Berscheid et al. and Miller et al. offers a hint as to what *simplification* means, we would expect the more neurotic and anxious group to dwell on chronic dispositions in characterizing others.

Funder presented all subjects, whether anxiety-prone or not, with a list of twenty-four trait terms (analytic, energetic, and so forth), with the instruction that a target person be rated on each of the traits *or* that the subject instead check "depends on the situation." Altogether, three kinds of target persons were rated: the subjects rated themselves, a close friend, and also a distant acquaintance. For every target person, the results showed that the explainer-subjects who tended to be stress-prone, anxious, lacking a sense of humor, and defensive employed significantly more trait terms and made fewer references to the situation. Just as in the Berscheid et al. experiment, the threatened individual tends toward simplification in explanation by ascribing permanent characteristics to the person.

Can these differences be called differences in perspective taking? Comparing the explanations given for the three different stimulus persons is informative here. When "taking their own perspectives," that is, when characterizing *themselves* through the twenty-four-item format, Funder's subjects referred frequently to situational factors. References to situations were less frequent when friends were characterized and still less frequent in the case of acquaintances. It is, then, fair to say that a relatively heavy reliance on trait-characterizations corresponds to neglect of the others' perspectives or at least to neglect of the others' perceived causes of their own actions.

This point is further underscored by White and Younger (1988), who asked their subjects to perform a self-characterization as well as a depiction of another person (usually a parent or sibling). The authors then broke down the two essays into specific components, to analyze how the self and the other person were depicted. Among the 18 subjects, a total of 64 traits were used in the self-depiction and 114 traits in the analysis of the other person—this much highly consistent with Funder's findings. Second—and here the differences are highly informative—the self-analyses contained many more references to short-lived psychological states, such as attitudes, feelings, and cognitions. For instance, feelings were mentioned a total of 227 times in the self-depictions but only 72 times in the other-depictions. Specific cognitions were mentioned 273 times in the self-characterizations but only 71 times in the other-characterizations. In short, and this time independent of the Easterbrook-derived control thesis, there is apparently a general tendency in explaining others' behavior to neglect short-lived, nonstable psychological states.

Frustration and Incompetence in Important Tasks and the Mode of Explanation

Within Easterbrook's terminology, we can examine one further research tradition that bears directly on the "naive" explainer. In a series of studies by Koller and Wicklund (1988) and Wicklund and Braun (1987), subjects were confronted with performances of varying difficulty. In one situation (Koller & Wicklund) subjects were asked to work anagrams, which were either soluble or practically insoluble. In addition to the difficulty of the task, extra pressure was placed on some subjects to perform well.

Once subjects had attempted their anagrams, they were requested to write a communication for the next subject, explaining "Which preconditions must a subject fulfill in order that the anagram task be solved?" Thus, the way was opened for subjects' giving technical descriptions of how to come to grips with the tasks, for characterizations of people who can solve anagrams, and the like. The results were in keeping with the findings of Funder (1980), but they also shed light on the workings of the performance-pressure variable. Subjects for whom the task was overwhelmingly difficult, and who were under high pressure, used a singularly high number of trait-terms in characterizing the performance setting and the ideal performer, such as "intelligent" or "persistent."

Highly parallel effects occurred in an experiment by Wicklund and Braun (1987), in which the dependent variable was "How often do you think about the traits of an ideal manager?" The combination of threat to competence and strong performance-expectations brought subjects to state that they spent more time thinking about performance-relevant traits. In addition, correlational studies (Wicklund & Braun) have shown that novices (i.e., people lacking skills in law or art) tend to depict the experts in those areas in terms of permanent characteristics. A reasonable summary statement of these several studies is that persons ill-equipped to perform but who feel pressure to perform well tend increasingly to think about performance in terms of the traits or physical qualities of the performer, and thus refer less to the actual details of the performance situation.

The Threatened Explainer: Toward Structure and Simplicity

The psychology of the explainer is not a rich, theoretically laden enterprise. The heretofore regularly cited literature on explainers has made exclusive reference to the simple thinking of the *everyday* explainer (see Wegner & Vallacher's "implicit psychologist," 1977) or to the "naive" or "implicit" personality theorist, who has ideas about how groups of traits should fit together (Bruner & Tagiuri, 1954; Rosenberg & Jones, 1972). Our purpose in this introductory chapter has been to look at theory and research that says something about the psychological variables underlying the tendency toward the simple, stable trait-package, "Case A" mode of explanation. And we have seen some hints: the authoritarian personality, described by Adorno et al. (1950) as experiencing a chronic threat to social status, is (in the language of the Adorno et al. scales) inclined to favor the simple, Case A variety of explanation. Variability in human behavior is ruled out, contextual subtleties underlying behavior are ruled out, and the behavioral direction is seen as being governed by strong, stable, traitlike forces.

The bridge from Adorno's work to the broad Easterbrook (1959) thesis is an easy one. In the language of Easterbrook, the person fraught with conflict, plagued by frustration, ego-threat, or other sources of strong emotion, has less cognitive capacity to attend to contextual details. The Easterbrook statement applies quite readily to the explainer, in that a number of research directions address the explainer's personal difficulties, incompetencies, conflicts, frustrations, neuroses, and the like. The sum of these research directions indicates a lessened perspective-taking capacity and an accompanying emphasis on explanations consisting of a concrete, stable portrait. The person whose ego is threatened, who is not capable of handling a performance situation, whose control is threatened (and the like) is inclined to characterize others' behavior in terms of permanent, overt qualities; the jump, or inference, to the psychological condition is thus left aside.

Notes

1. Rather than the traditional distinction between *states* and *traits*, the term *condition* of the organism is used here to refer to all that is intended by the state/trait terminology. Therefore, the central construct to which the theorist refers (i.e., achievement motivation, cognitive dissonance, anxiety, and so forth) is treated under the rubric of a *condition* of the organism. This simplification is introduced here to avert disputes regarding a trait/state distinction. Whether or not that distinction is justified theoretically is discussed in Allen and Potkay (1981) and also in Chaplin, John, and Goldberg (1988).
2. "Types A and B" in no way refer to types of explainers, but rather, to two different forms of explanation. The analysis of those who produce such explanations is undertaken in the following pages.
3. These differences between the three locations do not find a ready explanation in terms of intelligence or the like. If anything, the children from the socially isolated vicinity showed a *better* development in logical operations.

2
The Transition from Lacking Perspective-Taking into Theory

Wildly extrapolating, one could say that the research just summarized, which hints at reasons for a Case A mode of explaining, applies to scientists as well as to the everyday on-the-street scientist. One could start with the potential theorist with a graduate education in the social sciences, and then analyze the person's ongoing psychological traumas, psychological conflicts, and incompetencies in certain behavioral realms. If the person then elects to *theorize* in those realms,[1] we arrive at the simple conclusion that the theory (explanation) would tend to take the form of Case A, in which respondents are reduced to sets of traits or other stable characteristics and their complex perspectives overlooked.

Such wild extrapolations are of course wrong-headed, not because psychologists as a breed tend to be free of frustration, conflict, and incompetence, but because numerous other factors bear on the manner in which a psychological explanation is formulated. What are these other factors? Here we have to rely on expert sources—three in particular—to understand the difference between an implicit theory and a genuine scientific, psychological theory.

1. *Rosenberg and Jones (1972)* define an implicit theory in terms of its elements. One important element is the nature of the *category* the implicit theorist uses, whereby the category is built around physical features, race, values, traits, and the like. The second element in the implicit theory refers to the implicit theorist's *beliefs* about how certain perceived characteristics hang together (e.g., *creativity* and *spontaneity*). According to the distinction drawn by Rosenberg and Jones, an implicit theory is *implicit* because it is not formulated in a formal manner: "It is unlikely that an individual could make many of his categories and beliefs explicit or, given these basic elements, that he could organize them into a formal and parsimoniously stated theory of personality" (p. 372). Other labels for such nonformal theories are "commonsense," "lay," and "naive."

2. *Wegner and Vallacher (1977)* also take a stand on the relative sophistication of the scientific or professional psychologist, noting that the layperson is overzealous in ascribing stable essences to others in order to account

for their behavior. The professional or scientific psychologist is said to be more sensitive to the situational flux surrounding a target person's behavior and thinking.

3. *Sternberg (1985)* emphasizes the formulation side of theories, observing that the implicit theory usually exists "in the minds" of the implicit theorist but remains nonexplicated.

Looking at these three suggestions, we see that the explicit theory requires a certain sensitivity to the respondent's context (Wegner & Vallacher), as well as a formal or systematic formulation. While the meaning of *formal* is not spelled out by the experts cited here, we might well assume that they are referring to interworkings among variables. In any case, we are led to think that almost everyone possesses a number of implicit, not formally stated theories that neglect the differentiated background and other aspects of the respondent. The formal theorist (and the accompanying explicit theory) brings this kind of naive thinking to a higher, more systematic, differentiated plane. With this line of reasoning we would not suppose the scientific psychologist's efforts to be affected by control needs, by the personal need for a simplified Weltanschauung, or anything of the kind. But is this indeed the case? Let's have another look at Sternberg's (1985) portrayal of the explicit versus implicit theorist:

"Explicit theories are constructions of psychologists or other scientists that are based on or at least tested on data collected from people performing tasks presumed to measure psychological functioning" (p. 607). Thus, one critical criterion is that the explicit theory must have a certain empirical support or foundation; further, and perhaps all too obviously, the explicit theory must be communicated—usually written down and published. The starting points for both implicit and explicit theories are thus approximately the same, but they diverge at the points of locating data to correspond to the theory and of writing the theory down for mass consumption.

Commitment, Control, and Competition Enter the Picture

In an idealized scientific world the explicit or formal theorists would examine data relevant to the theory and communicate the theory widely, while remaining dispassionate regarding their involvement in the behavioral realm being studied. If theorists remain true to the depiction of Wegner and Vallacher (1977), they would retain their openness and differentiated view toward the respondents being studied. On the other hand, a commitment to a particular view of the human may well bring with it a number of psychological consequences. For instance, it is no secret that commitment to irrevocable action carries a built-in narrowness of thinking. The selective exposure tradition within cognitive dissonance theory (Brehm & Cohen, 1962; Festinger, 1957; Frey, 1978; Mills, 1965a, 1965b) and Kiesler's (1971) work on commitment point to the tendency of the committed person to reject information that is incongruent with the chosen course of action. One implication for the present is straightforward. If a person selects a trait-portrait out of the implicit realm of theorizing and makes it *explicit*, the theorist's resistance to incongruent information should thereby increase; that is, once the formal picture of the human is written and published, openness to contradictory information should decline.

Control assumes a very central role, now that we are speaking of a person who has taken an open stand regarding a certain portrait of the human being. Let's suppose, for instance, that a theorist has developed a theory of stubbornness, in which six facets of the stubborn person are pieced together into the "stubbornness" construct. This theorist thereby makes an open commitment to the position that the stubborn person-category embodies the characteristics "inflexible," "consistent," "unintelligent," "overweight," "masculine," and "stemming from very cold climates."[2] Given that having an explicit theory implies an active research undertaking (Sternberg, 1985), the theorist is committed to gathering data congruent with this verbally described picture of the stubborn person. This implies a definite *control need* vis à vis all potential respondents who can potentially be classified into the stubborn/not-stubborn system. Control means, very simply, that a person who is classified as stubborn must (with no or very few exceptions) also manifest lack of intelligence, masculinity, consistency, and having come from a cold climate. To the extent that this forecasted picture does not hold true in empirical reality, the theorist has lost control. In turn, the control need has definite implications for the manner in which the perspective of the respondent is neglected, as was spelled out in Chapter 1.

Competition now enters as the third element in this triad. As the number of psychologists in a certain subfield increases, so does the number of aspiring explainers. It is not clear whether the number of aspiring explainers increases linearly with the total number of active psychologists, or exponentially, but at a minimum large numbers of scientists working within one subarea of psychology should bring an increment in competition. Why competition? The issue is "Competition for what entity?"

Within psychology the entity has to be "the human mind and its functioning." This is the agreed-upon focus of research and theorizing efforts. But what happens when each of 100, or perhaps 1000 or 5000, research psychologists turn their attention to the human's complex functioning? If the psychologist's theoretical observations are based on the actual perspective of the respondent, then respondents will be studied in terms of their histories, both distant and immediate, and special attention will be given to perceptions, cognitions, habits, motivations, emotional tendencies, and the like. It is here that the problem begins.

These 100, 1000, or 5000 psychologists are competing for an entity that is in limited supply. Let's take a simple example. A starting point for many social psychology books is the remarkable (at that time—1951) demonstration of Asch, that people are susceptible to the influence of a unanimous opinion. The larger the majority, the greater the influence.[3] In exploring the psychological side of this relationship, two possible perspectives, or processes, were examined. First, subjects shifted their positions openly, even though they did not believe in this new position; second, the subjects became convinced by the majority, actually altering their perceptions (see Deutsch & Gerard, 1955). Psychologists looking at the first perspective in detail must focus on such factors as the subject's sensitivity to disapproval, the necessity of making a favorable impression, and the like (Jones, Gergen, & Jones, 1963). Psychologists who look at the second perspective in more detail must focus more on the several contextual factors, or dispositions of the person, that determine internalization of opinion change (Kelman, 1958; Snyder, Mischel, & Lott, 1960).

Once a few psychologists have tried to follow the course of these respondent perspectives, looking at them in detail, it becomes difficult for the next group (or generation) of psychologists, given that the next group is also interested in conformity issues. If the latecomers are going to say anything original about the respondents' personalities, perceptions, motivations, and the like, they will have to look carefully if they are to find components of the two or more perspectives that were overlooked. They are perhaps less likely to make a discovery.

Given that the fields of conformity, social influence, social learning, power, and others have become extremely popular areas of study, it goes without saying that the 5000 or more people studying these areas are confronted daily with an increasingly difficult, complex task. No matter which perspective they try to follow up, someone has already examined it; the room for original discoveries is scant. The fresh social scientist is then caught in a dilemma: The usual course of events for someone with a curiosity about human behaviors and their complexities is to follow one's nose, and to attempt to uncover in detail the multifaceted perspectives of the respondents. But one must first wade through the volumes of observations already existing and then attempt to chart the course of the respondents' perspectives, or psychological processes, in such a way that no single predecessor has ever done. If this effort fails, one's contribution is nothing more than a redundant observation, a replication.

This point can be distilled into the following observation. If the number of psychological processes that are readily discoverable is limited, then the number of possible theoretical statements is also limited. That a field or subfield has reached such a point is perhaps readily discernible by the sign of crises, in which basic research is abandoned ("it has all been discovered anyway") in favor of applications, or by the observation that the new theories all seem to be restatements of the classic theories.

Easterbrook's Thesis and the Scientist

An insuperable environment or task is an issue of the relationship between the individual's competencies or preparedness and the complexity of the entities that make up the task. The research cited in Chapter 1 (Berscheid et al.; Funder; Miller et al.; Vallacher; Wicklund, & Braun) focused on the individual-competence or threat-to-control side of this relationship. One reaches the same effect, that is, an insuperable environment, when the environment is adjusted in complexity. This was seen in the research by Koller and Wicklund as well as that by Wicklund and Braun.

If we translate the above to modern developments within certain empirical realms of social science, we have the following situation: the number of theories and models multiplies continuously, the amount of literature to be mastered increases as a logarithmic function of time, the complexity of statistical methods one should be able to use grows and changes, and the number of other scientists whose work is directly relevant to one's own is immense. The conclusion, therefore, is that we should expect an accompanying movement toward simplifying, toward neglecting the complexities of the respondents' perspectives, and a shifting away from consideration of processes that involve a conception of a changing, dynamic organism.

One can state this implication in terms of a control thesis. The modern psychologist concerned with complex human behavior is confronted with a lasting threat to control. So many processes of motives, motivations, perceptions, and cognitive mechanisms have already been examined that a newcomer should be reluctant to dive into such a confusing morass of psychology. Further, the more poorly trained one is, the more reluctant one should be. The alternative, implied directly by Easterbrook and subsequent researchers (Chapter 1), is to look for a simple, outwardly definable, and not so changeable entity. One becomes interested in the more fixed parts of human nature.

This orientation toward fixed, observable aspects has an important implication for the way in which the psychologist sets out to study the human. Rather than examining a phenomenon and asking oneself what hidden perspectives underlie that phenomenon, the psychologist is more inclined to focus on the manifest behaviors that respondents exhibit and on their other stable, overt qualities. The jumping-off point for one's theorizing is, then, not the search for the various perspectives of the people being studied, but instead a one-sided focus on the external and the stable.

But the idea must be carried a step further, following up on the preceding hypothesis regarding competition. A career or scientist-identity cannot be made simply by testing existing simplified characterizations of the human. Rather, the successful social scientist is seen as a creative, individualistic person, of whom it is said, "That is a really unique contribution." Fitting these two elements together—the tendency to (1) adopt explanatory modes that resemble our *Case A* and (2) simultaneously demonstrate one's uniqueness in relation to other contributions—we are led in the direction of a development that will be called the *zero-variable theory*.

Notes

1. A tongue-in-cheek hint at such a phenomenon comes from Jones (1964), who observed that because he wrote about ingratiation, he was repeatedly asked how he happened to become interested in that area.
2. Such theories were quite popular around the turn of the century, for example, in the works of the French sociologist de Lapouge (1896).
3. In the meantime the issue of numbers in the majority has received a still more differentiated treatment. Discussions by Gerard, Wilhelmy, and Conolley (1968), Latané (1981) and Schneider (1976) are enlightening in this regard.

3
The Zero-Variable Theory

The kernel of the zero-variable theory is a set of behaviors. In and of itself, there is nothing very problematic or objectionable about making a set of behaviors central in one's theorizing; it is what the theorist does with these sets of behaviors that is crucial. In the present context we focus on the classes of behaviors that are generally of interest to those studying complex human behavior—behaviors in social situations or with clear connections to social events.

Depending on their particular interests, theorists seek out groups of behavioral instances that seem to be related to each other. Thus, at the outset the theorist perceives certain similarities among several behavioral possibilities, such as "untalkative," "reticent," "unfriendly"; or perhaps "outspoken," "impulsive," "open." Nothing inherent in the sets of behaviors forces their selection for study; the selection process and perception of relevance within behavioral sets come from the theorist. One theorist might be highly restrictive, focusing just on "suicidal" and "self-destructive," while a second theorist might include all conceivable tendencies that can be labeled "active" (as opposed to "passive").

The next step in theorizing is the critical one; it is here that orientations diverge, with one theorist building a theory composed of psychological variables and another constructing a ripe zero-variable theory. What are the differences?

The one theorist inquires into the background perspective of the respondents who exhibit the behaviors in question, that is, into their perceptions, motives, motivations, latent tendencies of all kinds, and how these processes affect one another. Theorists who are guided by such respondent perspectives arrive at conceptualizations about the origin and the workings of certain psychological *conditions* (i.e., of perceptions, motivations, and other conditions).

A Theory with Variables: Achievement Motivation

A simple example: McClelland and co-workers Clark, Roby, and Atkinson (1949) began with an interest in entrepreneurial behavior, persistence, success-striving, and the like, but very quickly departed from the level of such behaviors and moved in the direction of the psychological perspectives of their respondents. In these background perspectives the researchers found certain patterns of child-rearing (Winterbottom, 1958), certain manners of self-expression (Aronson, 1958), and most important, sets of circumstances under which achievement motivation was maximized or minimized (Atkinson, 1957; Atkinson & Feather, 1966; McClelland et al., 1949). The central feature being studied became the respondents' *motivation* and accompanying perceptions. It could no longer be said that "entrepreneurial" behavior is simply a permanent behavioral tendency, which is perhaps related to very similar behavioral tendencies. Instead, the kernel of the theory became the *background* of the respondent, that is a certain psychological condition of the respondent (McClelland, 1961). This central condition—achievement motivation—was then found to be determined by several forces, some stemming from the respondent's childhood, others from competing tendencies (e.g., anxiety), and others based on the respondent's perceptions of the personal relevance and difficulty of the present task situation (Heckhausen, Schmalt, & Schneider, 1985).

Such a mode of psychological theory-building has important earmarks. First, the kernel of the theory shifts from the theorist's original interest in a behavioral instance to an underlying psychological condition. This condition (e.g., achievement motivation) is, in turn, a function of several psychological forces, belonging to the respondent's contemporary or historical background. Second, the human is regarded as *more* than the behavioral tendency in question. That is, the person is seen as being subject to psychological forces that come to bear on the central psychological condition. This means that the behavior with which one began (entrepreneurship, persistence, success-striving) loses its importance; it is simply one possible manifestation of the combination of psychological forces that stem out of the respondent's total perspective. Rather than a theory of the *entrepreneurial person*, the achievement motivation theory has become a notion that accounts for the occurrence of a variety of behaviors. Third, the respondent is no longer an everlasting *entrepreneurial type*, predestined to manifest entrepreneurial qualities. Rather, entrepreneurial behavior is one manifestation of the momentary workings of several aspects of the respondent's background perspective.

Such a theory can be characterized as one with *psychological variables*. The background of the subject is examined for variations in what is perceived, in relevant training, in what is learned, and finally in the extent to which achievement motivation is aroused. The psychological theorist is, practically by definition, one who does this kind of probing into the background variables that influence the dynamics of central psychological conditions. In the language of Lewin (1931), such psychologizing carries the name *Galilean*.

Creating a Zero-Variable Theory

Against the backdrop of achievement motivation thinking, the development of the zero-variable theory is easy to describe. The first and defining step is the theorist's continued concentration on the behavioral level, with attention directed *away* from the background of the respondent. In the idealized case of the zero-variable theory, the theorist has no idea of the respondent's background perspective, nor is he interested in exploring it. The theoretical statement, in any case, does not imply such an interest. This means that variables basic to a psychological condition—that is, to perceptions, motivations, and so forth—will not be incorporated into the theory. The beginning point of the analysis—the grouping of behavioral instances into a seemingly meaningful whole—is also the stopping point of the theoretical analysis. But what else? No one would try to argue that the mere identification of a cluster of behaviors is a theory!

The "something else" is the classification. The theorist groups together people who show this cluster of behaviors (e.g., suicidal, self-destructive), separating them from those who do *not* show such behaviors. This distinction between the "doers" and the "don'ters" then forms the kernel of the theory. The remainder of the exercise is a technical endeavor, which entails two deciding elements. First comes a continued concern with the behavioral grouping. How narrow or broad should the behavioral cluster be? Exactly how much should one explain? Can "hostile behavior" sensibly be placed together with "suicidal tendencies"? The second element is the act of categorizing, and it is here that the *person* of the theorist plays a major role. The theorist must locate or construct a device—a criterion or earmark—that successfully classifies all people into one or the other category. Such criteria need to be clear and visible. For many years the zero-variable theory classified people according to race (see Hilgard, 1987; Sorokin, 1928), gender, age, or similar criteria. For instance, de Lapouge (1896) put together a comprehensive system based on the deciding criterion of race, which divided humans into three categories: "Aryan," "Homo Alpinus," and "Mediterranean." In addition to spelling out the unique physical characteristics of each group, which served as the obvious means of categorizing, de Lapouge also went into great detail regarding each type's behavioral potential. The potential for great achievements, for dependence/independence, need for a strong government, energy, and other factors were woven into the tripartition.[1]

The deciding feature of such criteria is, of course, that they classify well, no matter whether they are based in race, geographical origin, or other overt qualities. If people grouped into one category *always* show the behavioral cluster, and those placed into the other category never show it, the classification device is said to be valid.

Going Modern: The Rational Method of Classification

A shortcut can be taken in these classification efforts. One can just use the behaviors to be explained as the criteria for assigning subjects to the two (or three) categories. Although the use of race, geographical origin, or gender might eventually lead the investigator to the formation of reliable categories, the categorizer can be more certain that the categorizing will operate as intended if the behaviors to be explained also serve the function of categorizing. This shortcut takes advantage of the "rational" approach to scale construction (Broughton, 1984), which means that the scale items are actually samples of the behavior that the scale is intended to predict (see Goodenough, 1949; Loevinger, 1957). The opposite of such a rational approach is the "empirical" method (Broughton, 1984), in which the classification criteria do not contain the behaviors that are to be explained. For instance, the items of the MMPI generally do not refer directly to the symptoms that are to be explained (see Loevinger, 1957), and similarly, racial or geographical criteria cannot point directly to the behaviors to be explained. Instead, such criteria are used as *signs* (Goodenough, 1949)— signs that the person so categorized will behave in line with the theory.

In implementing the rational approach to constructing a classifying device, the theorist can easily commit the error of assuming that all self-reports of the behaviors of interest (e.g., energetic, open, creative, spontaneous) reflect the trait acurately. We should emphasize two warnings here regarding this kind of assumption, these warnings being pertinent throughout the remainder of the chapters.

First, Meehl (1945) notes that the a priori piecing together of scale items requires "the assumption that the psychologist building the test has sufficient insight into the dynamics of verbal behavior and its relation to the inner core of personality that he is able to predict beforehand what certain sorts of people will say about themselves when asked certain sorts of questions" (p. 297).

Second, according to Loevinger (1957), "In principle, every trait of a person is represented in each of his actions. Some kinds of actions are such insensitive indicators of certain traits as to be worthless . . ." (p. 644).

The zero-variable approach is singularly insensitive to these kinds of reservations, because the dynamics of the person and the inner core of personality to which Meehl refers are of no immediate interest to the zero-variable theory. Within the several zero-variable schools covered in subsequent chapters, rational scale construction means nothing more than that respondents are trusted to report their chronic behavioral tendencies with fidelity and consistency. Accordingly the term *rational*, as used here, refers not only to the face-valid character of scale items, but also to the explainer's faith in the rational and honest self-descriptions of subjects.

The Competitive Aspect: Making One's Endeavor Unique

Once such a set of behaviorally pertinent items is put together, there is still a further step. The theorist is not content simply to predict what will happen; the uniqueness of his contribution must also be brought to the fore. In part, this can be accomplished by picking out a behavioral realm that no one has ever studied or by regrouping already-researched behavioral realms into a unique combination (e.g., "masculine gender role stress"; Eisler, Skidmore, & Ward, 1988). But still more important in establishing scientific identity is selecting the name for the classifying instrument. One method is to label the items, for instance, the "Smith Social Behavior Inventory" or perhaps the "Smith Inventory." More commonly, however, the set of scale items is given a label that the theorist calls a *construct*,[2] resulting in a term like "argumentativeness" (Infante & Rancer, 1982), "androgyny" (Bem, 1974), or "social competence" (Levenson & Gottman, 1978). The construct with which the theorist's name is associated appears to be novel, thus guaranteeing uniqueness. However, the result is deceiving: the "construct" in no manner stands for the psychological workings of the respondents who fill out the scale. Rather, the scale items consist of nothing more than the behavioral tendencies that are of interest to the theorist, and the so-called construct is simply a label for the combination of those items.

When Does It Become Theory?

No one would propose that the act of classifying, per se, constitutes a form of theorizing. Classifying has many different functions, including rendering the world less complex (Rosch, 1978); it also allows one to locate objects or people more efficiently (Anastasi, 1958; White, 1980). Classification is also important in experimentation, in that the effects of certain processes can be measured only by classifying people's responses, for example, into "morally mature" versus "immature" (Hoffman, 1977), or "attitude change" versus "no attitude change" (Hovland, Janis, & Kelly, 1953).

The question of when it becomes theory is best answered by observing what happens once a researcher has arranged to classify people into two groups. A number of subsequent steps inform the observer regarding the potential theorist's intentions: (1) an explicit characterization of the behavioral tendencies under scrutiny, (2) the technical perfection and further precision of the classifying instrument, (3) the attempt to demonstrate the uniqueness of one's instrument relative to competitors, and (4) the orientation toward totally reducing the person to one's own classification system, thereby ruling out alternative facets of the respondent. Although none of the explainers discussed in the next chapter uses the term *theory*, each of the zero-variable systems is promoted as something that "accounts for," "explains," or in some manner lays claim to broad groups of behaviors. Given the claims of each of these endeavors, the word *theory* is used here to capture the idea that the zero-variable theorist is oriented toward offering a singular account of a substantial range of complex human behaviors. Recent history has shown an acceleration in this type of theory-building, and our purpose in the next several chapters is to illustrate how the theorist goes about this task.

Notes

1. The reader may note that Sorokin (1928) issues a thorough critique of the de Lapouge position, pointing to inconsistencies between the alleged contents of the racially defined categories and the established empirical differences between those categories.
2. In the zero-variable theory one equates *construct* with a list of behaviors, disregarding its correct meaning (see Campbell & Fiske, 1959; Cronbach & Meehl, 1955; Loevinger, 1957; Meehl, 1945, 1978).

4
The Formulation of the Zero-Variable Theory

When we read about a "type" theory we seldom ask about its exact formulation. We are led instead to ask "What does the type do?" and "Is the type reliably different from other types?" However, if we were even minimally faithful to the philosophy of science introduction sections of our own text books, we would ask, "What are the interrelations among psychological variables that lead to the theoretically pertinent reactions?" In short, the reader who is confronted with a type theory is often asked to apply substandard criteria, and is not to expect an explicit, conceptual formulation entailing variables.

Since the zero-variable theory, also a "type" theory, has no variables, the theoretical statement is clearly not a formulation about the interworkings of variables. The focus of the theory is on the theorist's selected-out, categorized behavior tendencies; in other words, the "conceptual" statement of the theory is a listing of the behavioral tendencies in question. Let's look at this claim in the context of a small sample of such efforts:

Argumentativeness. Infante and Rancer (1982) have drawn a distinction between "argumentative" and "not-argumentative" behavioral tendencies. The theory is formulated as follows:

Argumentativeness is conceptualized as a generally stable trait which predisposes the individual in communication situations to advocate positions on controversial issues and to attack verbally the positions which other people take on these issues. The individual perceives this activity as an exciting intellectual challenge, a competitive situation which entails defending a position and "winning points." Feelings of excitement and anticipation precede an argument. Following an argument the individual feels invigorated, satisfied, and experiences a sense of accomplishment. (p. 72)

The individual low in argumentativeness is also described in detail, and is cast as the opposite sort of person, who avoids arguments and so forth.

Self-monitoring. Snyder's (1974) theoretical conceptualization is, as with Infante and Rancer, a listing of behavior tendencies: "concern for social appropriateness, sensitivity to the expression and self-presentation of others in social situations as cues to social appropriateness of self-expression, and use of those cues as guidelines for monitoring and managing self-presentation and expressive behavior." (p. 529) The low self-monitor, needless to say, does not display these tendencies.

Androgyny. According to S.L. Bem (1974) androgyny is a blend of masculine and feminine tendencies. Thus, the first step in the conceptualization is to define the respective tendencies of "masculine" and "feminine" types. This was accomplished by means of student raters; adjectives were generated that were thought to be relevant, then a list of 20 masculine characteristics and 20 feminine characteristics was finally agreed on. Some of the feminine qualities were empathic, warm, supportive, nurturant, and sensitive. The masculine qualities included tough, aggressive, pushy, independent, nonconforming, and athletic. These tendencies are the building blocks of the theory; the androgynous type is then quite easily defined as a blend of both masculine and feminine characteristics. In short, according to the theory the androgynous person is independent, sensitive, aggressive, and empathic.

Attributional complexity. The statement of the theory (Fletcher, Danilovics, Fernandez, Peterson, & Reeder, 1986) consists of seven tendencies that earmark the complex attributor (pp. 876–877):

1. Level of interest or motivation: "Attributionally" complex laypeople are said to be more curious about and interested in the whys and wherefores of human behavior.
2. Preference for complex rather than simple explanations.
3. Presence of metacognition concerning explanations, that is, a tendency to think about the underlying processes involved in causal attribution.
4. Awareness of the extent to which people's behavior is a function of interaction with others: attributionally complex people tend to notice and use information garnered from interactions to a greater extent than attributionally simple people.
5. Tendency to infer abstract or causally complex internal attributions. (One assumes that the tendency to infer abstract or causally complex internal explanations is associated with increased attributional complexity.)
6. Tendency to infer abstract, contemporary, external causal attributions.
7. Tendency to infer external causes operating from the past.

This characterization of the complex attributor is accompanied by two "hypotheses." The one hypothesis is that the seven components work together consistently, thus, "people who are more complex on one attributional dimension will be more complex on the other dimensions." The authors have thereby made explicit what is highly implicit in all comparable conceptualizations. The second hypothesis overlaps with the complex/simple distinction and is constituted by two further categories: women are said to be more attributionally complex than men.

In short, the theory consists primarily of the categories "complex" versus "simple" and "male" versus "female," with a certain amount of overlap between "complex" and "female." As in the formulations of argumentativeness and self-monitoring, a concrete list of tendencies constitutes the statement of the "theory."

Need for cognition. The original empirical treatment of "need for cognition" was by Cohen, Stotland, and Wolfe (1955).[1] At the time they regarded the need from the perspective of deprivation and implemented the concept without using a standard measure for the hypothesized need. In 1982 Cacioppo and Petty noted, "Surprisingly, there is no instrument available for measuring individuals' need for cognition" (p. 118), and in turn, they developed such an instrument. The theory underlying this scale, as formulated by Cacioppo and Petty, is somewhat more compact than those listed above: Those with a high need for cognition tend to *engage in* and *enjoy* thinking. In addition, it is said that "individuals of high rather than low need for cognition are more likely to organize, elaborate on, and evaluate the information to which they are exposed . . ." (p. 117).

The Commonalities of These Person-Characterizations

It is easy to see that the first step in the formulation is selecting a behavioral domain that the theorist intends to represent. The five examples given here vary considerably in their nature and scope; some are more socially oriented than others, some more oriented toward cognitive skills, some more elaborated than others. However, they share the following characteristics. Each one is nothing more than a list of behavioral tendencies or potentials. The argumentative person seeks out debating situations; the self-monitor tries to play the role that corresponds to the immediate social environment; the androgynous person shows sensitivity, empathy, and independence from social influence; the person with attributional complexity employs complicated explanations; and finally, the person with a high need for cognition engages in and enjoys thinking. Nothing in the characterizations points to variations in perceptions, motivations, or needs that might lie behind the overt behaviors that are listed.

All five of the formulations are silent on the issue of the origins of the types in question. We are evidently led to suppose that the people classified as argumentative, androgynous, and so on have always been that way. Thus, the characterizations are used as the starting point for research or application: one takes the characterization as it is presented, and then looks further to see what the person does (this point is treated extensively in Chapter 8).

Given that respondents are dealt with (via the categories) without the theorists' knowing what has preceded respondents' filling out the scale, we are led to think that their perspectives have been neglected or denied by the theorist. The only important thing about the respondents is their readiness to be classified as high or low, by means of devices that are discussed in the next chapter.

Another facet of the characterizations is interesting. In all of the characterizations the various behavioral tendencies within a category are regarded as mutually consistent. The theorist does not simply list behaviors that happen to be of interest; rather, it is assumed (highly explicitly by Fletcher et al., 1986) that the inhabitant of a given category is inclined to show all of the behaviors belonging to the category. In this sense each theorist postulates a kind of consistency theory, in which groupings of behavioral tendencies are said to hang together for any given person.[2] This is, of course, equivalent to what is commonly understood as "implicit personality theory" (Rosenberg & Jones, 1972), whereby the common person is said to link certain traits together.

An Exercise in Postulating Additional Theories

We have not gone far in detailing the modern zero-variable theory, but before proceeding, it will be good to show that *anyone* can coin such a theory. The Case A explanation, and thus the zero-variable theory, which reduces the human to a stable package of behavior tendencies, provides a simple alternative to theories that force the investigator to examine the respondent's background perspectives. This being the case, the formulation of a zero-variable theory should not be terribly difficult; the subjects in the threat-to-control conditions of Berscheid et al. (1976) and Miller et al. (1978) were working toward this goal, and so were the frustrated and incompetent subjects of Wicklund and Braun (1987) and Koller and Wicklund (1988).

Let's begin by listing some behavioral tendencies, and see how quickly the list turns into a theory. For example, we may postulate a category of people who are lazy, lethargic, slow, and phlegmatic; the opposite category would be energetic, full of initiative, and awake. This is the essence of the theory. To round out the theory, we need to label the list of behavioral tendencies. We can select "self-starting," a "construct" that does not yet exist in the literature. The positive appearing category contains "self-starters" and the opposite category "non-self-starters." The theory is perhaps important because this particular combination of tendencies has not yet been tried out, and certainly not with the "self-starting" label. The reader is assured that something new is afoot; a whole new arena of significant, complex human behaviors is about to be explained.

The Sternberg principle. The scientist will object that our theory is trivial, in that it is not accompanied by operationalizations or data of any kind. However, neither are the other five theories, at least not to this point. By Sternberg's (1985) definition, the theories we have summarized here, as they have been presented, are ostensibly nothing but *implicit* theories. The jump to the explicit theory is as follows: "Explicit theories are constructions of psychologists or other scientists that are based on or at least rested on data collected from people performing tasks presumed to measure psychological functioning" (p. 607). This transition from implicit to explicit cannot wait any longer. This brings us to the next chapter.

Notes

1. In fact, the idea was coined by Murray (1938), who was not subsequently cited.
2. A theory-relevant scale does not necessarily have to be "validated" through the demonstration of positive relations among the various behavioral tendencies listed. For instance, if a scale is designed around a dynamic model, there might be very good reason to expect *negative* relations among some of the behavioral possibilities. According to Loevinger (1957), "one dynamic structural possibility is that two particular manifestations of the same trait may be mutually exclusive or in a less extreme case, negatively correlated" (p. 668). For example, if one takes seriously the idea of need for cognition, it may well be that some people with a high need would adopt Route A (reflected in Item A of the scale) while others with a high need would adopt Route C (reflected in Item C of the scale). Each person satisfies the need, but neither person uses *both* Routes A and C consistently. Oddly, this very reasonable possibility is overlooked within the zero-variable formulation.

5
The Classification Device

This is the point at which the technical–psychological skills of the theorist–investigator must come to the fore. Two groups of people need to be created, thus two categories, with the one category *always* showing the one batch of tendencies (e.g., tending to think; enjoying thinking) while the other category always shows the opposite (i.e., not thinking, not enjoying thinking). One method of doing this is to seek out various obvious physical markers, until something is found—age, nationality, religious affiliation, sex, race, or physiognomy—on which one can build the two desired categories. Such a procedure has been followed in psychology and sociology, drawing on such demarcation criteria as geographical aspects or climate associated with a culture, not to mention race and religion (Hilgard, 1987; Sorokin, 1928).[1] These kinds of classification devices are called "empirical" (see Broughton, 1984), because their relationship to the behaviors of interest is an empirical question. That is, the leap from category criterion (race; geographical origin) to the behavior or thought patterns of interest is indirect. Similarly, the contents of certain well-known tests, such as the MMPI, the Strong Vocational Interest Blank, and the Humm–Wadsworth Temperament Scales, bear no obvious semantic relation to what the investigator would like to explain. The relationship between test content and the symptoms to be examined is established *empirically* (Meehl, 1945). But the *rational* approach has meanwhile taken hold in psychology and plays a central role in the expansion of the zero-variable school. Respondents are confronted with such statements as "I more often talk with other people about the reasons for and possible solutions to international problems than about gossip or tidbits of what famous people are doing" (Cacioppo & Petty, 1982, p. 120). Such a procedure assumes merely two elements: that subjects have cognitive access to the way they are inclined to behave, and that they are inclined to report in a way that is consistent with their behavioral inclinations. This is, in any case, the *rational* or *sampling* (Loevinger, 1957) approach to classifying people; the questions go right to the core of the behavior at hand. As a further example, one of the characterizations of the self-monitor in Snyder's (1974) theory is "concern for social appropriateness." If we look at the scale items used to categorize respondents, one of them reads, "When I am uncertain how to act in a social situation, I look to the behavior of others for cues" (Item 7). Or, turning to the argumentativeness theory of Infante and Rancer (1982), we should recall that part of the characterization had to do with the respondent's active approach of debating opportunities. True to the characterization, one of the items reads, "I enjoy a good argument over a controversial issue."

What determines how many such items are needed to classify people correctly? On this matter there is no uniform agreement. The smallest number of such items in a current zero-variable theory is 7, in a "public self-consciousness" measure from Fenigstein, Scheier, and Buss (1975). One also sees item lists numbering upwards of 30, as in the case of S.L. Bem (1974) and Cacioppo and Petty (1982). One cannot say that there is any uniform preference for a very small or very large number, but the items do in any case constitute an *elaborated* reflection of the person-characterization that we have called "theory" in the previous chapter.

What kinds of contents are found these items? For the most part one sees specific kinds of behavioral tendencies: Subjects are simply requested to indicate whether or not (or to what extent) that tendency applies to their own person.

Argumentativeness. If respondents claim to possess the following tendencies or characteristics, they tend to be placed into the high-argumentative category. Just to name three such tendencies: energetic when arguing, enjoy arguing about controversial issues, and able to do well in arguments. In parallel fashion, the respondent tends to be categorized as low-argumentative by assenting to such notions as the following: enjoys avoiding arguments, feels nervous and upset after having an argument, and happy to prevent arguments (based on Infante & Rancer, 1982).

Self-monitoring. One can gain membership in the high self-monitoring category by assenting to self-descriptions such as the following: puts on a show to impress others, does not always reveal one's true self, can tell a lie with a straight face. To be counted as a low self-monitor, the person assents to such characterizations as these: behavior expresses one's true inner self, doesn't change opinion to win others' favor, and is not good at improvisational acting (based on Snyder, 1974).

Androgyny. Unlike the other categorizations discussed here, the masculine/feminine categories underlying the androgyny category contain no negative examples; all of them are "socially desired" attributes. The respondent who assents strongly to both "masculine" tendencies (e.g., dominant, individualistic, masculine) and "feminine" tendendies (e.g., gullible, tender, yielding) will come to reside in the androgynous category (based on S.L. Bem, 1974).

Attributional complexity. People who are classified as "complex" are inclined to assent to propositions such as the following: it is important to analyze one's own thinking processes, analyzing the causes of people's behavior is enjoyable, and gives thought to the influence that society has on people. Similarly, respondents are classified as cognitively simple if they assent to the following items: doesn't analyze others' behavior, doesn't enjoy discussions about the causes of behavior, and prefers simple explanations for others' behavior (based on Fletcher et al., 1986).

Need for cognition. The high-need category is made up of such components as: is optimistic about mental abilities, is an intellectual, and prefers life to be filled with puzzles to be solved. Respondents are placed in the low-need category based on such criteria as the following: lays an issue aside once it becomes confusing, has problems in thinking within unfamiliar settings, and does not find abstract thinking to be appealing (based on Cacioppo & Petty, 1982).

Let's make some observations on these routes to classification. First, the reader sees that the "theory" cannot really be comprehended until the contents of the scale items are made apparent. The person-characterizations (see the previous chapter) are often rather sketchy, and one has to wait for the elaborated form of the characterization to grasp the kinds of tendencies the theorist has in mind. To be sure, when a theorist refers to a given category, a great deal is going on. For instance, Bem's androgynous person, who consists of all twenty feminine and all twenty masculine traits combined, encompasses forty different aspects. Needless to say, there is a good deal of redundancy within each of these elaborated lists, so that it would not be fair to equate the number of behavioral tendencies with the number of items.

Second, the reader might also note considerable overlap *between* the item sets. If we look at the first three scales, we see a number of items within each scale that refer to social competencies, a self-confident manner, and the like. In the last two scales we see a number of items that refer to various kinds of intellectual leanings. This means that different theorists are, in part, laying claim to the same territory. The extent to which this poses a problem is, in turn, a crucial part of the theory-building. These aspects are discussed in detail in subsequent chapters.

Third, each author proposes exactly one single scale as the appropriate categorization device. This will continue to be an interesting point in the development of the zero-variable theory and, as we will show later, has to do with the author's insistence on the supposed singular quality of the "instrument."

Fourth, one might note that the contents of the items are the sole basis for conducting research to test the theory. Thus, aside from the sketchy, minimal, or sometimes all-encompassing quality of the original person-characterization, the real jumping-off point for research, and determinant of the breadth of the territory to be claimed, is ultimately the contents of the scale items. Following is an example.

Cacioppo and Petty (1982) could perhaps have reduced their scale to the items "I think a lot" and "thinking is fun." People so categorized would then be expected to behave accordingly, thus, to register for philosophy and mathematics classes, to work crossword puzzles, to enter debates, and the like. The item "I am hesitant about making important decisions after thinking about them" (scored negatively) is a surprise entry; it seems to ask subjects not only about thinking, but also about hesitancy upon entering a decision. However, the fact that the authors have included this item in the categorizing device means that a certain decision-making facility is also expected from the favored category, that is, the high-need group. In short, by constructing a rather wide-reaching scale, the authors are able to capture more territory of complex human behavior. The important proviso is that all subjects inside the category behave consistently, in the sense of tending to show all the behaviors appropriate to the category.

Some Naive Questions

While the five theories illustrated here are presented by their authors as though the development of their respective scales would somehow follow "naturally" from an implicit chain of logic, the uninitiated reader automatically arrives at certain questions about these methods. The more central of these can be distilled into the following.

Why A Single Self-Report-of-Behavior Scale?

If the operationalization (i.e., the set of items) is intended to tap into a general disposition, or overriding behavioral tendency or complex (i.e., something psychological), then there must be more than one way to do it. If the explainer knows that the person being studied possesses an internal disposition, which in turn inclines that person to behave in set ways, then the only issue is that of tapping into the disposition. Conceivably one could do this with very few items (e.g., 7 items in Fenigstein et al., 1975), with a projective technique (see McClelland et al., 1949; Murray, 1938), or by means of external characteristics (race, nationality, gender). In short, if the theorist has come to terms theoretically with a certain kind of disposition, one need only *tap into* it. The only criterion for a good classification device is that it separate those who have the disposition from those who do not.

The approach taken by the zero-variable theory is, however, an extreme departure from the preceding reasoning. Instead of assuming that one device or another can tap into the disposition, the authors go out of their way to include *within* the categorization device all possible behaviors that are to be expected from people who hold the particular disposition. At first glance this approach seems to be overly cautious; further, one wonders why the theorist even needs to be a psychologist if the task is simply to list all of the actions the individual, classified as high or low, is likely to perform.

Staking out a territory. The question "Why a single self-report-of-behavior scale?" can be answered initially as follows. If zero-variable theorists are interested in claiming a certain behavioral territory as their *own*, with a kind of exclusive right to make pronouncements on or evaluations of those behaviors, it seems reasonable that the theorist needs to mark out the territory. There are not too many ways to do this other than through explicit reference to the behavioral forms that constitute this territory. If the theorist relies on an indirect classification device (e.g., projective test; race), and assumes that it taps a certain disposition, the theorist has no guarantee of any unique claim to the behaviors that might stem from the inferred disposition.

Let's try this reasoning out with a simple example. One theorist advances the concept of "argumentativeness" while a second theorist coins the concept of "assertiveness." Neither concept has any antecedent variables attached to it. Rather, the concepts are classification systems, constructed in the manner of those just presented. However, instead of using scales that refer to explicit behaviors, the respondents are classified according to projective tests. Respondents are shown simple pictures of social settings, in which various degrees of passivity/activity, aggressiveness, and so forth are imaginable. Subjects are then requested to write stories about the pictures. Theorist A scores the stories for "argumentativeness" themes, for instance, "How often does the central figure in the story argue?" Theorist B scores the stories for "assertiveness"—"How often does the central figure in the story push others around, get his way, and so forth?"

Based on the scoring of these stories, the first theorist divides people into high and low *argumentative* types: correspondingly, the second theorist divides the respondents into high and low *assertive* types. But then what? Obviously the next step is to predict behavior, but *what* behavior? The innocent bystander would simply watch the high and low argumentative types to see what they do. The high and low assertive types would be similarly observed. And it goes without saying that the two types would do a lot of the same things: many of the actions of the high argumentative type would have an assertive, aggressive, or strong willed character. And much of the behavioral repertoire of the high *assertive* type would have an argumentative, aggressive, or strong willed character. The naive observer would conclude that we are talking about the same person. Why employ two words for the same batch of behaviors?

To circumvent this problem the theorist must stake out the territory more carefully. Given that there are many competitors (explainers) for all facets of complex social behavior, the most sensible way to ensure the individuality of one's territory is to mark it off precisely, and highly literally, by indicating exactly which behaviors one wants to explain. These behaviors are then incorporated into one's scale and constitute the territory that becomes one's private theoretical domain.

Is the Collection of Scale Items Psychologically Relevant for the Respondent?

Subjects are given these categorizing devices with the implicit assumption that each behavioral dimension makes sense in terms of the subject's daily life, and also with the assumption that the subject is consistent with respect to the given behavioral tendencies. Such assumptions are highly questionable. For one, it is easy to document that subjects, particularly when describing themselves as opposed to others, are inclined to refuse to characterize their chronic tendencies if they are given the option of saying "depends on the situation" (see Funder, 1980; White & Younger, 1988; Wicklund & Braun, 1987). Second, a study by Sande, Goethals, and Radloff (1988) indicates that contradictory *self*-descriptions are more likely than contradictory *other*-descriptions. When respondents are presented with pairs of mutually opposing traits, they are likely to ascribe *both* of those traits to themselves. However, when *another* person is being characterized, there is a stronger tendency to iron out the contradiction. This pattern of findings upsets the view that the self-describer is constantly prepared to deliver a true and consistent self-characterization. Consistency is apparently greater when someone else is being described.

The originator of a list of behavioral tendencies can only hope that subjects' reactions to the items have their roots in deep-seated, chronic behavioral readinesses, but such faith is sometimes scarcely justified. Too many indications show that consistency in self-descriptions is simply an aspect of subjects' questionnaire behavior.

1. Knowles (1988) gave his 720 subjects a number of known scales (e.g., dogmatism, Rokeach, 1960), presenting the items in different orders for different subjects. The focus of his interest was the statistical reliability of individual items, in the sense of each item's correlation with the total test. His results were compelling: the *later* in the sequence of items that any given item appeared, the more it correlated with the total test score. An analysis of the phenomenon revealed that answers tended to become more polarized toward the end of the item sequence, and that this polarization was responsible for the increased consistency between late-appearing items and total test score. In short, the consistency here has nothing to do with actual behavioral potential; rather, subjects are simply more consistent in their answers as the test wears on.

2. In comparing subject samples of different ages and education levels, McFarland and Sparks (1985) find that consistency in self-reports increases as a function of both age and amount of university education. In short, the subjects' cognitive prowess appears to play a role in their answers, quite aside from whether the responses have any bearing on the behaviors they are said to represent.

3. Still more critical is an observation of Loevinger (1957). Let's

assume, along with the authors of the five scales described previously, that each scale does tap into a psychological construct, that is, a trait or a psychological disposition. For instance, if some individuals indeed chronically experience the psychological condition "self-monitoringness," then the presence of that disposition might well be reflected by high scores on at least some of the test items. However, this by no means requires that the subject be simultaneously high on all twenty-three of the items. According to the Loevinger (1957) observation, the presence of the disposition would lead individuals to act on that need or motive in particular ways, whereby *other* possible routes to acting on that need or motive would necessarily *not* appear. In short, the presence of a strong disposition will lead the person to act on that disposition in certain limited ways.

This problem has been addressed in part through statistical analyses that have found several different factors within scales such as the self-monitoring test (see Briggs & Cheek, 1988; Briggs, Cheek, & Buss, 1980; Nowack & Kammer, 1987). But the problem we address here goes one step further: if a person's self-monitoring disposition, need for cognition, or other characteristic is indeed an active psychological condition that impels action, then certain acts will come to the forefront and others will take a back seat (Loevinger, 1957). This simple observation has found very good support in research on cognitive dissonance (see studies by Götz-Marchand, Götz, & Irle, 1974; Walster, Berscheid, & Barclay, 1967) as well as in research on social facilitation (e.g., Cottrell, 1972; Zajonc, 1965) and aggressive drive (Frenkel-Brunswik, 1954). Thus, on the actual behavioral level, *some* of the behavioral tendencies must correlate *negatively* with one another. Otherwise one is not dealing with an active, psychological condition.

The zero-variable theory cannot take these problems into consideration, and perhaps for a very good reason. If a theorist uses a scale to mark out a particular, personal territory, one cannot very well say that the inhabitants of a category (high argumentative; high androgynous) use only *some* of that territory, and only *some* of the time. A definite claim to a given behavioral realm implies that the theorist's respondents behave in the specified ways chronically, and to the full extent.

It is important to note here that none of the zero-variable theories has any mechanism for describing when a person would be faithful to a given category and when not. To engage in that kind of analysis requires psychological variables, and these variables must come out of the background perspective of the people being studied. We are dealing here with theories with no variables, thus the respondents have no choice but to remain stable, consistent, full-fledged members of their categories. If their perspectives happen to be more complex than that, one simply forgets their perspectives.

Note

1. The physical criterion of biological gender also surfaces very frequently, for example, in the work of Bem (see Bem et al., 1976), Fletcher et al. (1986), and numerous other sources that are less central here.

6
Reducing the Human to a Categorized Empirical Essence

In a comprehensive analysis of the nature of explanation, Cassirer (1910) had something to say about the relationship between the explanation and the object being explained. He noted that certain classes of explanations— "Aristotelian" explanations—employed the character of the objects being explained in order to account for those objects' behavior or reactions. The starting point for Cassirer was the building of a concept, or category, in which the objects to be studied are grouped together, on the basis of their shared characteristics. As an example, he notes that cherries and meat could easily be placed within the same category; the two objects share the qualities of being red, juicy, and edible. To build such a category it is necessary to neglect all of those aspects that are not common to the objects, and for Cassirer, this is an important Aristotelian step toward shrinking the field for which one wants to account. The individuality, the quirks, and the contradictions inherent within each of the category members are thereby lost, since an object is a member of the category only insofar as it has qualities in common with other members.

The end result of Aristotelian classification is an ascribed *essence*, that is, a verbal concept that refers to nothing more than the sum of the commonalities of the objects within the category. In turn, this essence is reified and ascribed a causal role; the essence is then responsible for determining the total character of the objects within the category.

Lewin (1931), who picked up where Cassirer left off, translated this line of argumentation into the contemporary psychology of the late 1920s. It was Lewin's observation that the psychology of has day was dominated by an Aristotelian mode of thinking, which for him embodied a couple of telling characteristics.

Categorization was, for Lewin, the earmark of the Aristotelian approach to explaining. One of his examples: First the respondents are divided into age groups, perhaps children and adults, and their behavior is then explained on the basis of their category membership. Alternatively, people are divided into schizophrenic and nonschizophrenic classes, and their behaviors are accounted for by reference to the category.

The central problem, according to Lewin, was that the investigator who assigns someone to such a category thereby ascribes a *fixed essence* to that individual. That ascribed essence then supplants pertinent psychological forces acting on the person's behavior. This means that the person so categorized is no longer regarded as subject to the influence of pertinent psychological variables, that is, to background forces that lead to unique behavior or qualities. Instead, all that counts is that the individual behave in line with the prescriptions of the category in question.

As Cassirer, Lewin saw category-building as a process of abstraction:

Whatever is common to children of a given age is set up as the fundamental character of that age. The fact that three-year-old children are quite often negative is considered evidence that negativism is inherent in the nature of three-year-olds, and the concept of a negativistic age or stage is then regarded as an explanation . . . for the appearance of negativism in a given particular case! (Lewin, 1931, p. 153). . . . Quite analogously, the concept of drives, for example, the hunger drive or the maternal instinct, is nothing more than the abstract selection of the features common to a group of acts that are of relatively frequent occurrence. . . . Most of the explanations of expression, of character, and of temperament are in a similar state. (Lewin, 1931, p. 153)

Thus the *essence* that is ascribed by the theorist to the respondent is, in the words of Lewin, a set of behavioral tendencies that the members of a given category have in common.

Lawfulness as frequency. Given that the Aristotelian way of viewing things disregards psychological variables (i.e., neglects forces that lie outside the set of categorized behaviors), lawfulness in behavior can be construed only in terms of *frequency*. This means, very simply, that *frequency of occurrence* is equivalent to the lawfulness of what is observed. The more frequently the behaviors are exhibited by category members, the higher is the lawfulness.

Translated to the modern methods of categorizing, this means that all members of a given category must frequently (i.e., regularly) show the manifestations of category membership. They must all be regular and consistent with respect to their answers to the categorizing instrument and, of course, with respect to the behaviors that stem from their category memberships. All androgynous people must indicate on the questionnaire that they are "independent" as well as "sensitive"; they must also be prone to show "independent" and "sensitive" behaviors.

The idea behind the notion of *essence* is that objects are classified on the basis of common attributes. What they have in common, in psychology, is a set of reaction tendencies. Once they are so classified, they possess, by definition, the *essence* that is said to characterize category members (e.g., three-year-olds; people with a strong aggressive instinct). The essence, then, replaces an analysis of the psychological factors that act on indi-

viduals independent of their category membership. In the words of Cassirer (1910), the essence (equivalent to the common qualities of the category
members) takes over the role of determining the behaviors of the individuals within the category.

The Essence Is Forever

The reader will begin to object at this point. No reasonable, educated,
modern theorist would be so narrow as to propose that entire persons and
their behavior repertoires be reduced to a single category. Certainly the
theorist would admit that other aspects, external to the category, influence
the behaviors of interest. Even if a team of theorists places great stress on
the utility of their own category system for predicting independence, thinking, and other aspects, they would necessarily admit that there are other
sources of causal, relevant factors, and that a given person is not necessarily, under all circumstances, an "independent" person.

That may well be. But if so, then that would be the private opinion of the
theorist. The public statement or form of the published, formal theory
belies the theorist's flexibility, and to be sure, there is every reason to
think that Lewin's notion of an ascribed *essence* is a very real aspect of the
modern zero-variable formulation.

Without informing the reader about whether the behavioral tendencies
should be long-lived, or why, one of the first methodological steps is to
ensure that respondents answer the categorizing instrument the same way
over a time interval. One must see that the essence does not change. Let's
take a close look at how this procedure works.

Test–Retest Reliability[1]

In the case of Infante and Rancer (1982) the same respondents filled out
the questionnaire twice, with one week separating the testing sessions; the
subjects tended to fill out the questionnaire practically identically on those
two occasions (i.e., the correlation for the "approach argumentative situations" subscale was .87, while the correlation for the "avoid argumentative
situations" subscale was .86).

With the intervals varying between a week and four weeks, the other
theorists involved here have found similar test–retest coefficients. For self-
monitoring it was .83, for androgyny over .90, and for attributional complexity .80; no test–retest information is reported for need-for-cognition,
but it would go without saying that approximately the same results would
be found.

Why do the authors report such information? There is seldom, if ever, any explicit justification. The test–retest reliabilities are furnished, auto-matically, as though the scientific audience would have demanded them. An exception is found in the article by Fletcher et al. (1986). They ex-amined the reliability of their "attributional complexity" scale, noting that the high correlation confirms the "hypothesis" that the scale measures one construct—"attributional complexity" (p. 878). True to the remarks of Lewin, frequency (i.e., regularity of responding) is equated with lawful-ness, which in turn is equated with the appropriateness of the ascribed essence.

Why are the theorists systematically so stingy in their measurement of the basic tendencies over time? Seldom does one see an interval of more than one month between testings. Is there perhaps some fear that the high correlations will crumble as a result of hidden influences, methodological "noise," or other factors? Let's imagine the most disastrous possible case—the test–retest correlation, with a few weeks between testings, equals zero. It is guaranteed that the theorists we have illustrated here would discard such a scale as "unreliable." A new scale would be substi-tuted, new items found, the interval shortened to a more appropriate one week, and so forth. However, it would never be allowed that the question-naire responses themselves owe to psychological forces independent of the ascribed essence. The recognition of such forces is alien to zero-variable theorizing.

It will be helpful here to examine an alternative perspective. For in-stance, the test–retest reliabilities associated with the projective TAT mea-sure of achievement motivation are notoriously low, perhaps bottoming out at the value of .27 in a study by Winter and Stewart (1977) or .28 in Entwisle (1972). However, none of these values should be particularly astonishing, since it has already been shown that achievement motivation can be altered markedly as a function of subjects' immediately prior ex-periences (McClelland et al., 1949).

A related example: The original conception of need for cognition (Cohen, Stotland & Wolfe, 1955; Murray, 1938) regarded the need as a function of deprivation, and the empirical work by Cohen et al. sought to deprive subjects of a cognitive satisfaction or experience, with the expecta-tion that the need would increase. Thus, a theoretically true measure of need-for-cognition, as seen within the Cohen et al. context, should show considerable test–retest variability, depending on the extent of deprivation and satisfaction. This should apply only to the extent that the measure is indeed sensitive to the psychological construct *need*; more likely, however, the Cacioppo and Petty measure is little more than a list of behaviors, a point to which we shall return.

A further example: For particular ages, and in the course of particular learning contexts, a very *low* test–retest reliability in Fletcher et al.'s attri-butional complexity measure should be expected. The kind of hypothetical thinking to which they refer is a developmental product, that is, a complex interaction of genetic factors and learning context; one would not expect a child to show much of this entity at the age of seven, in comparison to thirteen or twenty years.

The point in these illustrations is simple: if the investigator were interested in psychological variables (deprivation, interference from competing needs, the outcome of critical learning experiences), the emphasis on test–retest reliability would be replaced with a view toward theoretically meaningful *changes* in the extent of what is measured. At the very least, one would arrange the test–retest procedure to eliminate the possibility of respondents' consciously trying to produce consistent patterns of responses over a period of a few weeks.[2]

Why Is the Consistent Essence Confined to Verbal Behavior?

An Aristotelian category is defined through the set of characteristics common to the category members. At the time of Lewin's writing, the primary, defining characteristics were generally fixed (gender; race), and consistency across time was, of course, no issue. The modern method of defining category membership is the rational-questionnaire approach, using the verbal level exclusively. But why? Given that the contents of the questionnaires refer to behavioral tendencies, the respondent's actual concrete behaviors should be at least as good a method of categorizing.

One of the few psychologists who have represented such an alternative approach is D.M. Buss (1985; see also D.M. Buss & Craik, 1981). In an illustrative study, respondents were asked to take three hours to indicate, for each of numerous acts, "how often you have performed it (if at all) *within the past three months*" (p. 172). The *acts* were such episodes as "I persuaded others to accept my opinion on the issue" (p. 179) or "I let another make an important decision for me" (p. 182).

Six months after the initial testing, respondents repeated the procedure, again indicating how frequently they had engaged in the particular acts. Buss then examined the consistency; that is, did engaging in the particular acts tend to remain consistent over a six-month interval? To be sure, the consistencies were greater than zero (as assessed by correlations), but compared with the test–retest reliabilities of S.L. Bem, Infante and Rancer, and others, the values were quite low. The average correlation was a mere .37. Assuming that stable dispositions underlie subjects' actions, those dispositions account for only 14 percent of the variance in the actions. It becomes understandable that the verbal approach, with rational questionnaires, is preferred for the building of categories. Through verbal responding, particularly when the time interval between testings is short, the theorist gains a picture of dazzling consistency across time—quite aside from what might bring this verbal consistency about (see Note 2).

Biological Origins

There are other reflections of the conception that "the essence is forever." If we examine carefully the theorists' ideas about the ultimate sources of their respective essences, we see a tendency to refer the essence to similar essences already existing. One very clear case in point is Snyder's (1987) analysis of the roots of self-monitoring:

People appear to be born with a biological-genetic predisposition to be high or low in self-monitoring. Then, over an extended course of socialization, small initial differences emerge in relatively restricted domains. They are then amplified and extended over time to eventually become the many and varied manifestations of self-monitoring . . . the social circumstances and life experiences that bring out the diverging self-monitoring orientations may be ones toward which people gravitate precisely because of their self-monitoring predisposition. (p. 153)

S.L. Bem (1974), in her analysis of the nature of androgyny, is very cautious in looking at antecedents and, in fact, offers no explicit suggestions as to the beginnings of these tendencies. Since there is a positive relation between biological gender and the masculine/feminine dimensions, we are led to think that the origins are supposed to lie in the genes, similar to Snyder's analysis. A similar reference to gender is seen in the attributional complexity notion of Fletcher et al. (1986). An allusion to the inheritance of the essence in question is also to be found in a zero-variable theory of Paulhus and Martin (1988), which they call "interpersonal flexibility." In forecasting the directions for their further work with the flexibility scale, they predict that "flexible parents beget well-adjusted children" (p. 99); that is, flexibility in the Paulhus and Martin sense is mentally healthy and appears to be inheritable.

Another zero-variable system (see a critique by Wicklund & Gollwitzer, 1987) consists of the categories "public self-consciousness" and "private self-consciousness." The scale to measure these entities stems from Fenigstein, Scheier, and Buss (1975). Buss (1980) attempts to trace the roots of these two categories. Interestingly, "privately" self-conscious people are said to begin as introverts whose introverted tendencies gradually ripen into private self-consciousness (Buss, 1980, pp. 246–247). In other words, the "privately" self-conscious person was "always that way," very similar to Snyder's (1987) portrayal of the origins of the high self-monitor, who begins with an inclination in that direction and then naturally ripens into a more definite category member.

Otherwise it is difficult to find explicit reference to the individual's origin of category membership, no matter which zero-variable theory we consult. In general, no reference whatever is made to the respondent's history, and if there is such reference, there is no indication that any particular factors brought the individual to be a member of the category. This way of approaching the individual's categorization follows quite directly from the observations of Cassirer (1910) and Lewin (1931). Individuals are grouped together in a category on the basis of some minimal number of shared attributes—in this case, their similar answers to questions about behavioral tendencies. All other facets of the individual are cast aside as irrelevant to the analysis of the category members. This being the case, it is understandable why the zero-variable theorist offers no analysis of the person's coming to be a category member. The whole analysis *begins* with the assumption that the person is already a member; factors extraneous to common membership criteria are no longer considered.

The Zero-Variable Theory: Single Operationalism and Positivism

The point of view of this book is that the psychologist's business, at least in complex social behavior, is to theorize about and research the person's perspective, that is, the person's psychological conditions (emotions, drives, perceptions). These psychological events are not visible to the naked eye. They are constructs—events postulated to take place within the person. The psychologist taps into these constructs by inducing them in different ways, measuring them in different ways, and looking at their postulated effects. Thus, the midpoint of the psychological analysis of complex human behavior is the inferred psychological event—motive, perception, and so forth.

In an elegant statement on the nature of psychological constructs, Campbell and Fiske (1959) note that a construct is ambiguous when there is only one means of operationalizing it. The idea is that a construct, as an overriding, internal psychological event, can be operationalized in many ways. If there were only one operationalization, the theorist may as well equate the psychological event with the empirical operationalization, and not bother with the construct at all. In other words, no inference from the operational or empirical level would be necessary. With one exclusive operationalization, the theorist can *see* the construct directly.

This point was made somewhat earlier by Cronbach and Meehl (1955). In discussing how one proves the validity of a psychological construct (e.g., anxiety), they warned that equating "anxiety" with a test that is said to measure "anxiety proneness" is an unsound procedure: the use of a single measure opens the way for almost unlimited alternative interpretations. "Academic aspiration" is noted by Cronbach and Meehl as one such alternative interpretation of a single anxiety measure. They note further that the test-maker must inquire into further kinds of evidence for the correctness of the interpretation. For instance, can one achieve similar results with alternative anxiety tests, or does the test reflect the direct induction of anxiety? Jessor and Hammond (1957), in a discussion of the Taylor manifest anxiety scale (1953), also remark that relying on one technique, or operationalization, to infer a theoretical process is a questionable business. Even Bridgman (1945), who carries the label "operationist," emphasized the importance of using several methods to infer a psychological concept.

Although practically all zero-variable theorists of complex social behavior cite or at least pay lip service to Campbell and Fiske (1959) and their predecessors, there is also widespread skepticism in psychology with respect to the inferring or postulating of "unseeable," untouchable" psychological events. As early as 1938, Murray observed that

The peripheralists have an objectivistic inclination, that is, they are attracted to clearly observable things and qualities . . . and they usually wish to confine the data of personology to these. (p. 6) Thus, for them the data are: environmental objects and physically responding organisms, bodily movements, verbal successions, physiological changes. . . . what characterizes them particularly is their insistence upon limiting their concepts to symbols which stand directly for the facts observed. In this respect they are *positivists*. (p. 7)

Using the term *tough-minded*, MacCorquodale and Meehl (1948) comment on a similar orientation toward the strictly observable: "one can still observe among 'tough-minded' psychologists the use of words such as 'unobservable' and 'hypothetical' in an essentially derogatory manner, and an almost compulsive fear of passing beyond the direct colligation of observable data" (p. 95). In a similar vein, Campbell and Fiske (1959) report that *single operationalism*, at least at the time of their writing, appeared to dominate psychology.

Thus, we see two qualitatively different standpoints. The one psychology, advocated by Campbell and Fiske (1959), Cronbach and Meehl (1955), and MacCorquodale and Meehl (1948), involves the postulation of mental or psychological events—nonobservable constructs—which are tapped into, accessed, or multiply operationalized by different techniques. This is the psychology that Murray (1938) refers to as conceptual rather than positivisstic: its terminology involves wishes, needs, and motives. The other standpoint, which is best described as positivistic or single operationalism, equates the psychological term with the single empirical event to which it refers. The level of thinking of this psychology is overt behavior, including verbal behavior, and perhaps also physiology.

The "Essence"

Applying these distinctions to our central problem, we can observe two things about the theories criticized here: (1) the "conceptual" language surrounding the theories refers entirely to visible, observable events (i.e., to the behaviors as listed in the scale), and (2) the theorist allows no operational definition, other than a home-grown scale, of the "construct." It follows that the zero-variable theory is another case of positivism, or single operationalism. The *essence*, that is, "androgyny," "self-monitoring," "argumentativeness," "need for cognition," or "attributional complexity," always *sounds as* though it would be a psychological construct, that is, an inferred psychological event that would be operationalizable in many ways. But it is nothing more than a title for a single list of behavioral tendencies. In every case the theorist is cautious, not entrusting psychological terms with an independent existence. The name given to the list of behavioral tendencies could just as well be changed to "List of Behaviors in Area X." By the criteria of Bridgman (1945), Campbell and Fiske (1959), Cronbach and Meehl (1955), Garner et al. (1956), Jessor and Hammond (1957), Meehl (1978), and Murray (1938), one sees only *exclusion* of psychological constructs.

Lewin (1931) foresaw this discussion of positivism in psychology with his comment that the "drive" concept can easily be equated with the features common to a group of acts. What he had not foreseen was a more extensive form of positivism, rendered possible by the modern technique of rational scale-construction.

Notes

1. Independent of its questionable character in zero-variable theory construction, one should also note that test–retest reliability has its legitimate place in test construction.
2. In principle, the idea behind reliability checks is to see whether a particular psychological condition can be measured on different occasions by the same instrument or by techniques that to some degree differ from one another (e.g., alternate-form reliability). This being the case, the investigator wants to be sure that test answers are attributable to the *psychological condition* in question, and not to other, more trivial factors. For instance, a high test–retest reliability may be a simple result of the recall of previous responses or, at a minimum, the recall of the pattern of earlier responding. This obvious point implies that one could obtain a high test–retest reliability even when the psychological condition of the subject has already ceased to exist. However, this point is seemingly meaningless within the development of the zero-variable theory. Consistency is highly valued, aside from the psychological reasons underlying it.

7
Proving the Uniqueness of One's Own Categories

We are two steps along toward the complete zero-variable theory: First, a behavioral catalog is put together in which the several behavioral forms are said to hang tightly together; second, the respondent's category membership is viewed as the single cause of these behaviors. But now we reach a point that is much more decisive for the *scientific activities* of the theorist: the category system must be shown to be unique.

The first chapter took a brief look at the switch from naive or *implicit* theory to *explicit* theory. The shift may be regarded as a commitment, on the part of the theorist, to represent publicly a certain picture of the human being. This commitment in turn is accompanied by a desire to exert control over the respondents who fall within the boundaries of the theorist's human portrait. If the respondents do not behave in accord with the portrait, the theorist loses control.

In addition to commitment and control, a third element — competition—can easily become a by-product of formulating an explicit theory. The entity to be accounted for is in short supply when one considers that numerous, perhaps thousands, of would-be theorists are trying to claim theoretical ownership of a certain domain. The result of such competition, aside from neglect of competing views of the human, is the effort to mine out one's individuality. The theorist's portrait of the human must stand out from others' claims to complex human behavior.[1]

A unique name for the categories is a small aspect of this search for uniqueness; far more important, and much more time-consuming, is the effort to show there is no overlap between one's own categories and those of others. In modern parlance this activity is referred to as proving the "discriminant validity" of the categorizing instrument; it works in the following manner.

First, a false reading of Campbell and Fiske (1959) is the basis of much of this discriminant validity activity. The critical passage from Campbell and Fiske reads "Tests can be invalidated by too high correlations with other tests from which they were intended to differ" (p. 81). Thus, respondents fill out the theorist's scale (e.g., self-monitoring) as well as another scale (e.g., masculinity/femininity). The theorist notes that self-monitoring is *not supposed* to be the same as masculinity/femininity. The correlation between the two is then computed, and if the correlation is low, the discriminant validity of theorist's *own* measure is said to be assured. Of course, it is assumed that the theorist has a clear idea about which other tests are not supposed to correlate with his own.

The passages of Campbell and Fiske (1959) that are not taken to heart are those on *con*vergent validity. The idea is that one should be able to assess a construct by means of more than one method. Insofar as one's construct is reducible to one solitary measuring device, the validity of the construct remains in question (Campbell & Fiske, p. 101). The implication is quite clear. If the kernel of the theory were a psychological condition (e.g., the construct *achievement motivation*), then there would be several ways to operationalize it, and perhaps even induce it, as McClelland (1961) and co-workers (see Heckhausen et al., 1985; McClelland et al., 1949) have shown. On the other hand, if the kernel of the theory is nothing but a list of behaviors, it is nonsense to speak of an alternative way of assessing it. One does not operationalize behaviors.

In practice, when we look at the modern zero-variable theories, this means the following:

First, the theorists have no clear idea of what other classification systems should and should not correlate with their own category systems. Generally they try to show that their own systems correlate with *no* other categories. When this does not work out, they refer to the significant correlations as instances of *con*vergent validity and label them as "moderate." The issue of discriminance is then dropped.

Second, other category systems are brought forth for the discriminant validity test in a *prestige* order. The theorist is interested in showing discriminant validity with respect to scales or other categorization criteria that are known, famous, highly recognized, and employed in everyone else's discriminance analyses.

Third, it will also become apparent that the total number of other classification devices picked for comparison with one's own device varies greatly from theorist to theorist. In the following, these points will come to light through a look at the exact manner in which the uniqueness-striving efforts are undertaken.

Argumentativeness

The discriminant validity exercise as undertaken by Infante and Rancer (1982) involves correlating the scale with certain "behavioral choices." The subjects were asked to indicate the attractiveness of four different activities: (1) debating, (2) delivering a public speech, (3) watching and rating TV programs, and (4) conversing with other students about goals in life. The idea, according to the authors, was to show that the scale relates particularly to the desire for argumentative-type activities, and not to communication per se. To be sure, the people who scored highly on the argumentativeness scale evidenced no special propensity to want to watch or rate TV programs or simply to participate in a conversation. But they did express an interest in public speaking and debating. In short, the argumentative person is not simply predisposed to communicate, but shows a desire for a very specific form of communication. Aside from this brief exercise, Infante and Rancer report no further discriminant validity calculations. The situation is, however, quite different when we examine our other four examples.

Self-Monitoring

The self-monitoring scale, whether composed of eighteen or twenty-five items, is said to reflect a person's propensities to lie, act, please others, and the like. In Snyder's language, the high self-monitor is a person with certain chronic tendencies, and the question surrounding the discriminant validity exercise is, "Might not such an individual be identified equally well by existing measures of related psychological constructs?" (Snyder, 1979, p. 92). Translated into methodological language, this question becomes, "Might not such an individual be identified equally well by existing scales (or classifying devices) that carry other names?" The discriminant validity exercise then entails finding out whether the person "identified" by the self-monitoring scale is also "identifiable" by someone else's scale. The scales or other classifying devices that are then brought into the picture are known, prominent, and frequently used in zero-variable theorizing literature. The list begins with "need for approval" and ends with "birth order."[2]

What are the results of this discriminance analysis? According to Snyder (1987, pp. 27–28), his scale shows meaningful correlations with *none* of these other classification systems. At this point the reader might ask a number of naive questions about this kind of procedure: (1) Why stop with twenty-two other classification systems? Isn't something missing? (2) What is the content of those other classification schemes? That is, is there overlap between the items of the opposing scales and the items of the self-monitoring system? Why were these particular scales chosen? One does not immediately see the relevance of these classification sytems for the behavioral tendencies listed in the self-monitoring scale. (3) Finally, what would the theorist have done had there been a high overlap between his own scale and an alternative system? The conclusion would have to have been, "An existing classification system identifies the person equally well. Therefore, the self-monitoring scale is superfluous and will have to be discarded." Fortunately, this does not seem to have happened, at least in Snyder's report (see Note 2).

Androgyny

Two classification systems were central in the discriminant validity exercise of S.L. Bem. As with Snyder, a burning issue was the classification "social desirability," and similar to Snyder's report, the correlation between androgyny and social desirability was reportedly "near zero." The other discriminant validity exercise is somewhat unique to the work of Bem; the attempt was to ensure the singular quality of the Bem scale within the context of existing measures of masculinity/femininity. Two alternative measures were drawn into the discriminant validity analysis—masculinity/femininity measures from the Guilford-Zimmerman Temperament Survey and from the California Psychological Inventory. The correlations between the Bem scale and each of the others were computed; they were reportedly quite low, and Bem concluded "the fact that none of the correlations is particularly high indicates that the BSRI is measuring an aspect of sex roles which is not directly tapped by either of these other two scales" (1974, p. 160). Again, the reader can ask (1) Why not use more scales? (2) Are the items of the opponent scales really so different from those of the Bem scale? (3) What could have been done, had the correlations been high?[3] In addition, a fourth question now arises: given that the predecessors of the Bem scale also carried the name masculinity/femininity, should we not expect a good deal of overlap between all of the scales? (see Campbell & Fiske, 1959). Or is Bem defining a type of "masculinity/femininity II" that has heretofore been neglected? We will return to these questions below.

Attributional Complexity

Fletcher et al. (1986) began in the same manner as other zero-variable theorists, focusing on popular classification systems that were to be differentiated from their own system. Thus, social desirability was again in the center of the analysis, followed by intelligence and internal/external locus of control. Social desirability was measured by the usual measure devised by Crowne and Marlowe (1964), intelligence by the American College Test scores, and locus of control by the Rotter (1966) scale. Just as in the preceding theories, we see that the discriminant analysis was successful: "As predicted, the discriminant correlations were all nonsignificant" (p. 880). Quite remarkably, Fletcher et al. find a correlation value of .36 in comparing their own scale with the Cacioppo and Petty (1982) need-for-cognition scale. How do they handle this instance of overlap? Does the failure of discriminant validity make their own categories superfluous? Not in the least. Instead, this correlation turns out to have been predicted yet of no great consequence: "However, the moderate size of the correlation suggests that the two scales measure different, albeit overlapping, constructs" (p. 880). The same kind of reaction to a significant correlation (with the CPI) is seen in Bem (1974), as well as in most other zero-variable discriminance analyses. The ideal is a perfect pattern of zero correlations with all other measures, but as soon as a disturbing correlation arises it turns out to be "sensible" but not debilitating. (The reader dare not ask what the borderline between "sensible" and "debilitating" would be. On this point there is no comment in the zero-variable literature.)

Need for Cognition

Disregarding any concerns about social desirability, Cacioppo and Petty proceed directly to two other scales. The one is cognitive style, which, they argue, is to be discriminated from need for cognition. Cognitive style was then assessed by the Embedded Figures Test (Witkin, Dyk, Faterson, Goodenough, and Karp, 1962). The other construct to be ruled out was test anxiety, as assessed by Sarason's (1972) measure. Just as with the preceding theories, the discriminant analysis exercise was successful; the correlations between the authors' own scale and these two alternative scales were quite small.

Alternatives to the Usual Discriminant Validity

The five discriminant analyses here are representative of modern and current zero-variable accounts of complex social behavior. The approach is to locate known, established classification devices, usually scales, and show that answers to one's own scale do not correlate with answers to the alien scale. But why is this approach taken? Encroachment on one's behavioral territory could be handled in other ways, such as the following.

Looking At the Items

A semantic analysis of the items would be highly informative regarding the amount of potential overlap between two "constructs." Rather than beginning a discriminance analysis on the basis of the prestige of competing scales, the investigators could simply determine whether they have repeated formulations that already exist in other classification systems. To the extent that there are repetitions, the redundant items in one's scale could then be eliminated to ensure its uniqueness. An interesting case in point is a contrast between two scales of self-consciousness; one by Paivio, Baldwin, and Berger (1961) and the other by Fenigstein, Scheier, and Buss (1975). Although Fenigstein and colleagues (see also Buss, 1980; Carver & Scheier, 1981) have conducted numerous discriminant analyses on behalf of the public self-consciousness scale, they have failed to include the Paivio scale in their analyses. Had they done so, they would have discovered on inspection a remarkable overlap in the nature of the items. There is a good

TABLE 7.1 *Autonomy* According to Murray (1938): Statements in Questionnaire

1. I am unable to do my best work when I am in a subservient position.
2. I become stubborn and resistant when others attempt to coerce me.
3. I often act contrary to custom or to the wishes of my parents.
4. I argue against people who attempt to assert their authority over me.
5. I try to avoid situations where I am expected to conform to conventional standards.
6. I go my own way regardless of the opinions of others.
7. I am disinclined to adopt a course of action dictated by others.
8. I disregard the rules and regulations that hamper my freedom.
9. I demand independence and liberty above everything.
10. I am apt to criticize whoever happens to be in authority.

From Murray, H.A. (1938), *Explorations in Personality*, p. 158. Copyright 1938 by Oxford University Press. Reprinted by permission.

deal of similarity between the seven items of the public self-consciousness scale and the six items of the older Paivio et al. (1961) scale. Characteristic of the older scale were "I am bashful with most strangers," "I often wonder what others think of me," I often worry about what people think of me," "Other people can hurt my feelings easily." Among the items of the newer scale (Fenigstein et al., 1975) are "I'm concerned about the way I present myself," "I'm self-conscious about the way I look," "I'm concerned about what other people think of me," "I'm usually aware of my appearance."

Such obvious semantic overlap alone should be adequate to bring theorists to abandon their claim to the territory in question, and to retreat to unclaimed areas. Alternatively, one can adopt the route of failing to refer to the earlier scale.

The same potential problem applies to any of the scales that are central here, for instance, to the self-monitoring scale. One would examine an existing list of behavioral tendencies, taken from earlier measures, and look at the item overlap. An interesting illustration comes once again from Murray (1938), this time from his "autonomy" dimension. The items, shown in Table 7.1, are in many cases quite close to negatively formulated self-monitoring items. For instance, Item 3 depicts a person who acts contrary to others' wishes, Item 4 refers to arguing with people who are in authority positions, and Item 5 ("I try to avoid situations where I am expected to conform to conventional standards") would also have made an ideal (negatively scored) self-monitoring item. Quite aside from which of the ten items we examine, one can see the portrait of people who *do not* try to please others in their presence. It appears that the self-monitor has already been defined by Murray, as the opposite of the autonomous person.[4] We see no references to the Murray scale in any of the self-monitoring literature.

The overlap with the self-monitoring items is even more salient in Murray's (1938) *deference* questionnaire (Table 7.2) with such items as "I

TABLE 7.2 *Deference* According to Murray (1938): Statements in Questionnaire

1. I am capable of putting myself in the background and working with zest for a man I admire.
2. I see the good points rather than the bad points of the men who are above me.
3. I accept suggestions rather than insist on working things out in my own way.
4. I am considered compliant and obliging by my friends.
5. I often seek the advice of older men and follow it.
6. I give praise rather freely when the occasion offers.
7. I often find myself imitating or agreeing with somebody I consider superior.
8. I usually follow instructions and do what is expected of me.
9. In matters of conduct I conform to custom.
10. I express my enthusiasm and respect for the people I admire.

From Murray, H.A. (1938), *Explorations in Personality*, p. 155. Copyright 1938 by Oxford University Press. Reprinted by permission.

am considered compliant and obliging by my friends" or "I often find my-self imitating or agreeing with somebody I consider superior."

The Fletcher et al. (1986) notion of attributional complexity also has its predecessors, that is, previous category systems that have been left out of the picture. The central quality of the person in the "better" Fletcher et al. category is an openness to complex, behind-the-scenes explanations. The items refer to thinking about underlying processes, the power of the social situation, and the internal, psychological state of the person. This same kind of category has been formulated, in reverse-worded form as an "in-tolerance of ambiguity" scale, by Martin and Westie (1959). Among the eight items of the scale are "There are two kinds of people in the world: the weak and the strong,""There is only one right way to do anything," "You can classify almost all people as either honest or crooked." A comparison with the items of the Fletcher et al. scale reveals a decided overlap.

It is not necessary to repeat this exercise with the other scales dealt with here. We may simply observe that the procedure of looking at the exact contents of the territory claimed, however that territory is labeled, is neglected. This selective avoidance of the contents of other scales follows directly from the premise that the zero-variable theory strives toward establishing its uniqueness, toward possessing a unique territory. Commonality of items with other theorists threatens this claim.

Comparing the Labels

Even when the previous approach is neglected, one certainly expects theorists to heed competing categorizing devices that carry the same label as their own. At the same time, we see that this must be threatening, for the presence of other instruments with similar or identical labels results in one of the following:

1. Not acknowledging the other's existence. This has already been discussed in the context of the Fenigstein et al. (1975) "self-consciousness" scale. A very similar self-consciousness scale was never cited. It is the same with Cacioppo and Petty (1982) whose "need for cognition" category bears an unmistakable semantic similarity to Murray's (1938) "need for understanding," whereby Murray's questionnaire items ("I am rather logical and coherent in my thinking"; "I enjoy reading books that deal with general ideas") bear a striking resemblance to those of the modern need-for-cognition questionnaire. The Murray scale seems to have been over-looked by Cacioppo and Petty, who state that: "Surprisingly, there is no instrument available for measuring individuals' need for cognition" (p. 118). Needless to say, we also see no discriminance analysis with respect to the twenty Murray items.

2. *Proving that one's own categorizing device defines the label ("construct") better than do the competing categorizing devices.* This approach is illustrated by Bem (1974), who, after comparing her own androgyny scale with two other approaches labeled "masculinity/femininity," concluded that her own "measures other aspects of sex roles." By this reasoning, it does not really matter if several people lay claim to the same territory, using the same term, as long as the measures of the term do not correlate with each other. We see a similar approach in the analysis of "flexibility" by Paulhus and Martin (1988). In their view, certain other categories— namely, androgyny, high self-monitoring, the California Psychological Inventory (CPI) flexibility scale, and Leary's (1957) adjustment scale—all deal with flexibility. Then, having made up their own relatively complex flexibility scale, they proceed to show that the other measures do not correlate with it very highly: "The first step in validating the FFI [the Paulhus and Martin scale] was to demonstrate adequate discriminant validity-. . . . the FFI loaded on a factor separate from the other flexibility measures" (1988, p. 99).

Comparing the Psychological Perspectives of the Respondents

In the zero-variable theory there is never any systematic comparison between the psychological condition postulated and alternative psychological conditions. A simple illustration suffices here. Infante and Rancer (1982), in referring to the "construct" argumentativeness, do not consider how other theorists might characterize the psychological states, orientations, motives, drives, perceptual styles, and so forth that could underlie the act of arguing. One does not have to look very far to locate theoretical statements that obviously have a great deal to do with argumentative, debating, give-and-take behaviors. For instance, the motivation to win an argument can derive from circumstances that threaten the integrity of one's belief (see Schachter, 1951). Thus, uncertainty about one's own opinion should be one possible component of the argumentative person's psychological background. Such comparisons, which necessarily are drawn on the level of an inferred, psychological condition (i.e., the respondent's perspective), accompanied by systematic variables, are not found within the realm of the zero-variable theory. This theme is addressed again in Chapter 10 on alternative explanations.

Summing Up the Zero-Variable Discriminance Analysis

Taking the preceding in reverse order, and adding the usual discriminance analysis to the list, we see four possiblilities for attending to the similarities between the behaviors one wants to explain in one's own category system and the behaviors that are already claimed by other systems:

1. Look at the similarities/differences in *psychological* content.
2. Give attention to systems that carry the same or similar labels.
3. Compare individual items within the classification devices.
4. Make the usual discriminance analysis.

Of these four possibilities, the first and third are *never* undertaken, and with the second, we see only that the theorist tries to minimize the apparent similarities between his and competing systems. Thus, the primary route taken to identify the uniqueness of the territorial claim is the statistical comparison, the correlation between one's own scale and a highly limited list of other scales. Given that the criteria for selecting these competing scales have more to do with their general prestige than their a priori overlap, one wonders whether these discriminance analysis efforts should be accorded any scientific value at all. They are highly selective, they refer only to the verbal level, and one gets the strong impression that the impetus behind them is to prove one's uniqueness, To be sure, given the theoretical work of Fromkin (1970, 1972) and Tesser (1980, 1986), we *should* expect these kinds of uniqueness-strivings. The apparent competence of the theorist who has made a commitment to a certain worldview, in this case to a given portrait of the human, depends heavily on the individuality of that portrait. The psychological basis of the theorist's engaging in these kinds of discriminance analyses is perhaps more compelling than the scientific outcome of these discriminance endeavors.

The Confrontation with Threatening, Alien Categories: When Positive Correlations Turn into Validity

No matter how carefully other category systems are selected, in the hope of demonstrating no overlap, the theorist cannot always be successful. Sometimes the facts become plain; certain overlaps with one's own categories are scarely avoidable. When the theorist is brought to acknowledge such overlaps, the solutions offered are interesting, indeed. Two of them are noteworthy, and the second ("validity") is worth some extra attention.

The Avoidance Solution

The zero-variable theorist stands the risk that all conceivable categorizing systems might overlap with the personally chosen one. One universal way to cope with this threat is avoidance, particularly of categorizing systems that are (or were) not current at the time of the particular zero-variable formulation. For example, none of our zero-variable examples mentions Murray's (1938) rich system of scales, nor is there any significant reference to the classic personality work of Cattell (1965) or Eysenck (1953). Further, nonquestionnaire methods of classification are not drawn into the discriminance analysis, perhaps surprisingly, in that stable physical characteristics of respondents provide potentially reliable indicators of differences between categories (see Sorokin, 1928).

The Misuse of Validity as a Solution

The validity of a psychological construct is shown through the use of different empirical approaches to that construct (Cronbach & Meehl, 1955). The investigator allows the theory to point the way toward operationalizations that should set the construct into motion, or tap into the construct— and, important for Cronbach and Meehl, one can speak of a valid *construct* only when there is converging empirical evidence for its functioning. The zero-variable approach treats the validity concept quite differently. The central activity is the *discriminance* analysis; this is undertaken to show that all pertinent comparisons (correlations) are minimal. Should one's own scale be shown to correlate, however, with an alien scale, this finding (a nuisance from the zero-variable point of view) is then dealt with by labeling the correlation "convergent validity," "concurrent validity," "construct validity," or something of the kind, never with an eye toward the correct sense of these concepts as illuminated in Campbell and Fiske (1959) and Cronbach and Meehl (1955). How does this step of the zero-variable theory function?

First of all, an ugly correlation arises—let's say a value of .40 between the theorist's own scale and some competing scale. Clearly this is no basis for claiming the two are different. The theorist then surprises the reader by announcing that the relationship between the two scales was *expected*, *hypothesized*, or something similar, and also, that it proves the *validity* (construct validity, concurrent validity, or some other kind of validity) of his classification device.

On those rare occasions when physical features of the respondents are correlated with the scale, the process is usually similar. An instance of *no* correlation proves that the scale is not simply redundant with gender, race, or age; yet when the correlation becomes high enough, it suddenly turns out that the scale "should, theoretically," have something to do with gender, race, or age. We might have a look at this flow of thinking in concrete cases.

Argumentativeness

Infante and Rancer (1982), in a "concurrent validity" analysis, report correlations between their measure and several other scales pertinent to communication (e.g., the Mortensen, Arnston, & Lusting, 1977, Predisposition Toward Verbal Behavior Scale). The obtained correlations were noteworthy (e.g., .45, .32, .35, .22). In the language of the authors, "all correlations were significant, in the slight to moderate range." (p. 77). Thus, such "slight to moderate" overlapping between scales supports the validity of the argumentativeness scale.

Interestingly, one of these correlations (.22) was actually lower than a value that was subsequently used to prove *discriminant* validity ($r = .23$). Here we see a hint that the authors are treating the mathematical side of psychology somewhat loosely: a relatively strong correlation (.23) is used to show that two things are *different* from each other, while a slightly weaker correlation (.22) is used to show that two things *resemble* each other. Taking this logic a bit further, one would welcome correlations of over .90 for discriminant validity, while correlations around .00 would demonstrate *convergent, concurrent,* or *construct* validity. If the reader is confused at this point, we can develop the confusion further.

Self-Monitoring

Despite Snyder's (1987) insistence that the correlations between self-monitoring and numerous other scales are negligible, a certain shyness scale is drawn upon for proof of the validity of the scale (pp. 20–21). The shyness scale stems from Pilkonis 1977, and the correlation between that scale and self-monitoring is $-.16$ (Pilkonis, 1977). Citing this latter finding, Snyder lists it among the various other validity-indicators.

Interestingly, the Pilkonis (1977) study also shows a correlation between self-monitoring and extraversion—a healthy value of .32. Extraversion, however, is regarded by Snyder (1987) as *not* "meaningfully" associated with the self-monitoring concept (1987, p. 27).[5] Thus the reasoning followed by Infante and Rancer (1982) is repeated, this time with more boldness: a correlation of $-.16$ shows *overlap* between two constructs (i.e., self-monitoring and shyness), while a value of .32 demonstrates that two constructs (self-monitoring and extraversion) are *non*overlapping.

The reader should be thoroughly confused. Obviously the theorist can have it both ways. Sometimes a case of overlap between the theorist's scale and an enemy scale is denied, that is, relegated to the status of "not meaningful"; the alternative solution is to consider such correlations as "friendly" (i.e., validating).

Given that S.L. Bem (1974) does not appeal to cases of scale-overlap for validity, we will move directly to Fletcher et al. (1986).

Attributional Complexity

Under the title "convergent validity" Fletcher et al. report a correlation between their own measure and Cacioppo and Petty's (1982) need-for-cognition measure ($r = .36$). Within the context of their discussion of this evidence for validity, they note, "However, the moderate size of the correlation suggests that the two scales measure different, albeit overlapping, constructs" (p. 880).

Need for Cognition

Cacioppo and Petty (1982) make less use of this "validity" device, but an interesting commentary is to be found in a discussion of *discriminant* validity. They note a correlation of .19 between a cognitive style measure and their own measure, with the annotation: "as expected, based on the constructs that each is thought to tap, a significant but small correlation was found . . ." (p. 123). The reader is baffled! Does "small and significant" prove the discriminant, or the convergent, validity? On the other hand, they have no reservations about reporting a correlation of .48 between intelligence and their own scale; it turns out to have been predicted.

Adding Public Self-Consciousness to the Collection

The convergent versus discriminant validity exercise is also well developed in Carver and Scheier (1981), in which various correlations with the public self-consciousness measure are said to evidence convergent validity. One of them involves a sociability measure, where the r value is .22. Once again, minimal relationships with other scales are welcomed as evidencing validity.

The abuse of the *validity* concept lets the theorist off the hook. Should a correlation with an alien scale threaten, and not be swept under the carpet as "negligible" or "not meaningful," the correlation magically acquires the quality of bequeathing one's own scale with validity. But there are limits to this strategy. The alien correlation is not allowed to be too high—reflected in the constant reference to "low to moderate, but significant correlations." Nowhere among our several examples is there a case of the theorist's admitting to a *high* correlation; high correlations make one's own categories superfluous.[6]

Not All Alien Categories Are Threatening: A Social Comparison Phenomenon

It is enlightening to look more closely at the kinds of categories that are drawn into discriminance analyses. They are invariably competing scales, and almost always rather contemporary. But what about subjects' behavioral styles, or fixed physical characteristics? These are also very fine category designators. Interestingly, almost all relations between one's own scale and behavioral styles or physical characteristics of respondents seem to be welcomed, as a kind of validity. Infante and Rancer (1982) find birth order to be a meaningful accompaniment of argumentativeness, Snyder (1987) views the overlap between self-monitoring and overweight as sensible, Fletcher et al. (1982) as well as S.L. Bem (1974) see gender differences as overlapping meaningfully with their scales, and Cacioppo and Petty (1982) regard a very strong overlap with occupational status as a kind of validity. This brings us to an unavoidable implication regarding the psychological impetus behind these many discriminance-and-validity exercises.

Uniqueness on Ego-Relevant Dimensions

The preceding review indicates that competition for territory takes place only with competing categories that (1) are also scales and (2) are well-known and recognized in the contemporary personality/social literature. Thus, not all categorizing systems are included in the competition, to be rejected or "discriminated." And interestingly, category systems that are noncomparable with one's own are not actively discriminated, but rather welcomed as a kind of proof of the goodness of one's own system. Thus, a contemporary, frequently cited system (e.g., social desirability; masculinity/femininity) must at all costs be discriminated from one's own categories; overlap is not tolerated. On the other hand, a healthy overlap with birth-order, occupational role, gender, or overweight is regarded in a positive light. One finds overlap with such noncomparable categories to be good—as showing the applicability, validity, or meaningfulness of one's own system.

This entire endeavor is highly reminiscent of the social comparison processes described by Festinger (1954) and elaborated on by Tesser (1980, 1986). One of Festinger's central observations was that competition accompanies comparability (Hoffman, Festinger, & Lawrence, 1954). If a subject's ability is within the same range, and on the same dimension, as another's ability, competition ensues. If the subject and the other person are completely noncomparable, there is no subsequent interest in competition. This line of reasoning is an apt description of the discriminant analyses just reviewed.

But the analysis can be carried a step further, implementing Tesser's

(1980, 1986) theory. If another person is not comparable, thus not ego-threatening, but at the same time highly competent (e.g., well-known), a certain identification with that person is to be expected. Translated, this means that if theorists find overlap between their own categories and another set of well-known categories (e.g. birth order), with low comparability, they welcome the association with that other set of categories. The preceding review indicates very strong support for this derivation from Tesser's analysis. One need only count: how often does a theorist admit to overlaps with another, contemporary scale (competitor), and how often does the theorist claim overlap with a category system that is *not* a scale?

The Zero-Variable "Theory": A False Accusation?

In the course of showing how the zero-variable system develops, the term *theory* has been applied freely, as though all of the authors dealt with here label their categorization systems "theories" and all the theorists say they are "explaining" behavior. In fact, the words *theory* and *explanation* are exceedingly rare. We could dispense with those terms but still retain the meaning of what is intended by the zero-variable approach.

The term *theory* has been used because each of the theorists in the preceding examples tries to deal with a given realm of behavior in an exclusive manner. The theorist picks out a behavioral territory and tries to *do something* with it. If the sole purpose of the endeavor were simply to describe the behaviors within that territory, then we would be dealing simply with the modest aspiration of predictive validity of scales (see Cronbach & Meehl, 1955, p. 283), in which the predictive character of the scale stands in the forefront and not the interpretation. But this is not the case. If prediction were the sole purpose, theorists would then not be interested in eliminating competing systems and would not refuse to examine the predictive power of their own systems relative to others.

Rather, the uniqueness-striving of the zero-variable theorist testifies as to the interpretive intent: the idea is to interpret, label, explain, account for, deal with, or bring under one's own umbrella a specified territory of human behaviors. It is for this reason that we have used the term *theory* to refer to the zero-variable endeavors. One could, of course, implement categorizing systems for entirely different purposes, such as finding additional operationalizations of an existing theoretical concept. Taylor (1953) constructed her anxiety measure with this intent, as an alternative operationalization of the Hullian drive construct (see Jessor & Hammond, 1957). McClelland and colleagues (1949) pieced together the TAT device for achievement motivation, deriving the techniques from Murray, as one possible operationalization of the motive. They also developed others (see McClelland et al., 1949; McClelland, 1961). This use of multiple measuring instruments serves the broader purpose of construct validity.

Or one can also be content with a simple predictive validity (Cronbach & Meehl, 1955), in that one is interested in finding some criterion, index, or scale from which a particular behavior or facet of the person can be predicted. As such, one would allow other predictive devices to exist.

But striving toward uniqueness is not the final step of the zero-variable theory-construction—there is one more phase that follows. The behaviors listed in the scale are assumed to be reflected on a more "behavioral" level. This brings us to the next chapter.

Notes

1. Theoretical analyses of the bases of such striving for uniqueness are found in Brock (1968), Fromkin (1970), Synder and Fromkin (1980), and Tesser (1980).
2. A healthy list of competing scales or other categorizing devices is presented by Snyder (1979, 1987) as "not correlating meaningfully" with the self-monitoring scale. These others include need for approval, Machiavellianism, extraversion, locus of control, inner-directed versus other-directed, field dependence, self-esteem, hypnotic susceptibility, neuroticism, trait anxiety, repression–sensitization, achievement anxiety, need for cognition, intelligence, academic achievement, religion, public self-consciousness, private self-consciousness, social anxiety, the clinical scales of the MMPI, socioeconomic status, and birth order. While one should not question the theorist's own judgments about what kinds of correlations are meaningful or not meaningful, one cannot help but notice others' reports of pertinent correlational analyses. One of these is a finding by Cheek (1982), who reports a correlation of .45 between the self-monitoring scale and the public self-consciousness scale.
3. A glance at the correlations with competing scales evidences suspiciously high values. Among the values (that are not "particularly high") is a correlation of .50.
4. The overall picture of the so-called self-monitor is reminiscent of Piaget's (1932) and Kohlberg's (1980) portrayal of the morally underdeveloped individual. The dependence on the approval of the immediate group and the absence of cross-situational consistency in matters of values and moral judgments are the defining features of the person whose cognitive development or social atmosphere has not led to a mature, autonomous mode of fuctioning. Perhaps not surprisingly, none of the self-monitoring–related discriminance analyses gives any attention to measures of moral development, such as measures by Rest (1976, 1980).
5. Also in Snyder's (1987) "not meaningful" list is the correlation between self-monitoring and public self-consciousness—the value of .45 reported by Cheek (1982).
6. Crowne and Marlowe (1964), whose social desirability scale is the starting point for most zero-variable discriminance analyses, view these kinds of discriminance–convergence exercises much differently. Having embedded their social desirability concept within a theoretical network, they do not see the necessity of proving zero overlap between their scale and all other categories. For instance, a value of $-.67$ between their scale and defensiveness was welcomed (see Crowne, 1979, p. 172), for good theoretical reasons.

8
Replacing Hypothesis-Testing with "External Validity"

The concept of a scientific hypothesis implies that the scientist is dealing with a questionable idea, thus one that needs to be tried out. The idea might read, "increased drive will enhance performance of dominant responses," or "response persistence will be enhanced by intermittent reinforcement," or "high achievement motivation produces a preference for risks." All such statements are notions about the relationships among psychological *variables*. The psychological variable is not equivalent to behavior but instead, part of a person's perspective—that is, an attitude, cognition, habit, emotion, arousal state, motive, or similar quality. "Drive," "habit", and "achievement motivation" are thus constructs that refer to the person's perspective, to a process inside the person, and to the way in which these variables fit together in the theory. As further examples, cognitive dissonance theory states that the more the volition involved in a decision, the greater the experience of dissonance, and Easterbrook's (1959) cue-utilization theory postulates that "the more the arousal or emotion, the narrower is the perceptual frame."

Such statements are actually *subjunctive*. One says, "A *should*, according to the theory, lead to B," or "If Variable M is raised to its highest level, then Variable N will no longer have an impact on the dependent variable X." These statements refer not to a factual, behavioral level, but to the conceptual level—to the organism's perspective, in our present language. The study or experiment is thus the attempt to operationalize these subjunctive or hypothetical connections on the level of objective reality.

Need for Cognition as a Psychological Construct

Let's take a simple example of a hypothesis regarding a certain kind of need, namely, the need for understanding or need for cognition (Cohen, Stotland, & Wolfe, 1955; Murray, 1938). Viewing the issue in terms of a dynamic drive theory, Murray notes, "An edifice of logically interarticulated concepts is the end situation which satisfies and quiets the tension" (1938, p. 224). Cohen et al. (1955) talk about the cognition-need in a similar manner, referring to the background of the individual in terms of blocking the satisfaction of the need. They propose, as a prologue to their experiment, that an ambiguous, hard-to-comprehend situation will frustrate the need for cognition, produce negative affect, and also lead to efforts to structure the situation to increase one's understanding. It is clear what one must do to examine this hypothesis: the more that individuals can be shown to be deprived relative to their needs, the more they will be frustrated and then tend to seek out cognitive structure.

This example refers to hypothesis-testing and is intended as a point of contrast. In the following it will become apparent that the procedure for the zero-variable theory is free of such hypotheses. It will also become evident that the subjunctive flavor is lacking entirely in zero-variable thinking: all speculation about results contrary to one's expectations is left aside. It is assumed a priori that the expectation must necessarily hold.

External Validity

This is the crucial step in the theorist's making a zero-variable theory out of a classification scheme. Seldom is the term *hypothesis* used in this context, even though this is the stage at which studies are set up to see what kinds of behaviors stem from the classification system. And why not "hypothesis"? The reason lies in the manner in which the scientific study comes into being.

The core of the zero-variable theory is a list of behaviors, with no specification of the variables that might be related to those behaviors. They simply *exist*, as they are listed in the scale. Further, their inclusion in the scale is based on the assumption that they are congruent with each other. The research effort is a small, highly cautious step beyond the scale, assessing whether or not subjects do, in fact, show the behaviors in the scale. Different theorists have different names for this cautious step: "convergent validity" (Infante & Rancer), "construct validity" (Snyder), "external validity" (Fletcher et al.), "predictive validity" (Cacioppo & Petty), "criterion validity" (Paulhus & Martin), and "construct validity" (Carver & Scheier). Thus, the scientific enterprise of the zero-variable theory now consists of three major elements: (1) the original statement of the theory, which amounts to a listing of broad behavioral tendencies, (2) the listing of those same tendencies in more detailed form within a scale, and (3) the observing of the actual enactment of those same behaviors. This three-element approach to psychological science is shown in Table 8.1.

By now it should be evident why a hypothesis is not necessary. There is nothing hypothetical, or subjunctive, about the step from theory to re-

TABLE 8.1 Building and Testing Theory Within the Zero-Variable School

1. *The theory*: A number of mutually consistent-appearing behavioral tendencies are listed as the characterization of a given type of person.
2. *The scale*: Those same behavioral tendencies are elaborated into specific scale items.
3. *External validity*: The same behavioral tendencies are observed on a more behavioral, nonscale level.

search. The theorist's implicit hope is that subjects will be consistent, that is, the person who claims to be assertive will in fact show rough or imposing behaviors. In the language of Lewin (1931), the idea behind these research endeavors is that the person who is assigned to a category will be true to that category, in the sense of consistently manifesting the characteristics of faithful category members. Let's see what this looks like in actual research.

Argumentativeness

In one of the "validity tests" reported by Infante and Rancer the subjects' reactions to an argumentative situation were examined. Subjects were led to think that they would have to engage in argumentative discussions with someone, and then they simply gave their liking ratings for the anticipated situation. Quite in line with predictions, the scale scores correlated (.36) with liking for the argumentative situation.

What about consistency? If we look at the argumentativeness scale, we see that the liking measure (i.e., behavioral measure) was indeed in keeping with some of the item formulations (e.g., "I enjoy a good argument over a controversial issue.") Common sense tells us we could hardly expect anything other than consistency, given that the content of the relevant behaviors is explicit in the items. But we will pursue the issue again later. What do other zero-variable theories look like in the realm of external validity?

Self-Monitoring

It has been found, for instance, that (1) high self-monitors are described by peers in a way that matches the self-monitoring characterization, (2) good actors have high values on the scale, (3) high self-monitors are adept at simulating emotions, and (4) self-monitors are inclined to deceive others. Once again, these behavioral manifestations are true to subjects' self-descriptions of their own behavioral tendencies. Consistency between scale contents and behavior is the criterion of good research.

Androgyny

The androgynous person, who constitutes the most interesting category in the S.L. Bem system, possesses a number of traits that appear, at face value, to be mutually contradictory (e.g., assertive and yielding; self-reliant and gullible). The idea is, however, that the androgynous person will be generally sensitive to situational demands, and will show either the feminine or the masculine reaction, depending on what is appropriate. This kind of reasoning led Bem to such behavioral measures as the readiness to show nurturant behaviors when given a baby to play with (Bem, Martyna, & Watson, 1976) or the ability to withstand social influence (Bem, 1975). Thus, with the proviso that the androgynous person waits to see what the situation calls for, the research program is the same as those of Infante and Rancer (1982) and Snyder (1987); the behaviors that are explicitly located in the scale are then observed.

Attributional Complexity

In a study that looked at the external validity of the attributional complexity scale, Fletcher et al. (1986) asked subjects to choose from different kinds of causes for particular events. For instance, in explaining why "Sue is afraid of the dog," subjects were given the option of naming a disposition explanation, circumstance-oriented explanations, or some combination of these, the latter being designated by Fletcher et al. as a "complex" attribution. True to the expectations, the correlation between scale score and actual complexity of the attributions was .31. In the words of Fletcher et al., "The more complex the subject, the more likely he or she was to choose the complex causal attribution" (p. 882). Interestingly, Fletcher et al.'s explanation for the results falls well within the "simple" end of their simple-to-complex continuum. Subjects who choose complex, environment-plus-disposition explanations are "explained" in terms of their membership in the complex, or desired, category.

These results reflect no more than a rudimentary consistency. For example, Item 9 of their scale was worded, "I have found that the causes for people's behavior are usually complex rather than simple." One would suspect that this one item, taken alone, would also correlate quite highly with the overt choice of complex explanations.

Need for Cognition

Cacioppo and Petty (1982) draw a distinction between two ways of construing *need*. One is a tissue deprivation notion, which clearly refers to the theoretical reasoning of Cohen et al. (1955). According to this view, a deprivation or frustration plus emotion precede the person's seeking cognitive structure. The other approach, according to Cacioppo and Petty, is "statistical," that is, need is treated in terms of likelihood or tendency. In turn, one sees how this second conception of need is then realized: *Need* is fully reduced to the Cacioppo and Petty scale, and its antecedents—the deprivation, frustration, and negative affect to which Cohen et al. refer—vanish from consideration. The psychological analysis of need turns into a reduction to a list of behaviors, a so-called statistical conception.

How does one test this system? The first study compares the scale scores of two groups: university faculty members and workers. The faculty sample was found to score much higher on the scale than workers. Why should this be? If we look at the scale items it is evident that such differences between status groups are a foregone conclusion, for example, "I prefer watching educational to entertainment programs," and "I am an intellectual." In short, a certain congruency between the scale and "occupational behavior" is assured a priori.

But what happened to the psychological construct *need*, as referred to by Murray (1938) and Cohen et al? If we take that construct seriously, we should perhaps assume that the workers must be frustrated, not having much opportunity to act on their need for cognition. Therefore, their need should be *higher* than that of professors. But the construct has vanished. All that is important is that the contents of the scale be reflected, in a congruent manner, on the overt or behavioral level.

Another validity test in the Cacioppo and Petty work looked at the relationship between scale score and enjoyment of a complex task. A simple task was defined as the circling of all 1s, 5s, and 7s, whereas the complex task involved circling all 3s, all 6s preceding a 7, and every second 4. In keeping with the contents of the scale, the people low on the scale preferred the simple task over the complex one, while the opposite was true for those high in the need. The consistency is thus apparent. Behaviors that are listed in the scale are also observable in overt behavior. People who say they like complex problems do, indeed, show a preference for complex problems.

Flexibility

Paulhus and Martin (1988) perform a validity exercise that is common among zero-variable endeavors (see Snyder, 1974). Acquaintances of the respondents are asked to provide flexibility ratings. If these are congruent with subjects' self-ratings, a certain validity—in this case "criterion validity"—is said to be attained. The raters—friends, acquaintances, or family members—were asked to rate the respondent on the following dimensions:

Deals well with social situations
Avoids certain situations
Adjusts easily to new social situations
Is likable
Acts inappropriately for the situation

The correlation between these ratings and subjects' own flexibility scores was .44. Is this validity? Paulhus and Martin (1988) say yes, but one has trouble in bringing this kind of validity into agreement with the notions of Campbell and Fiske (1959).

Public Self-Consciousness

The seven item "public self-consciousness" scale has been related to a host of behavioral manifestations. Most of these have to do with subjects' social dependency (see a critique by Wicklund and Gollwitzer, 1987). Perhaps characteristic of these studies is a correlational finding by Fenigstein (1979), showing that people in the "high" category are particularly vulnerable to rejection from others. A reading of the scale makes it clear that the results were a foregone conclusion, assuming that subjects were prepared to be consistent with their scale answers.

The Open Triviality of the Rational Approach in Zero-Variable Theories

Nicholls, Licht, and Pearl (1982) wrote a critique of such exercises as these, under the title, "Some dangers of using personality questionnaires to study personality." They argued that knowledge is hardly advanced, nor is the reader surprised, to learn that masculinity (dominance, independence) is positively correlated with dominant, independent behavior. To be sure, the kinds of consistencies that are examined in studies such as the preceding are striking in their redundancy, but this owes to the manner in which subjects are classified. The *rational* method of scale construction allows subjects to place themselves into categories through self-descriptions, the problem being that the self-descriptions are the same behavioral tendencies that are to be studied. A cynic would describe the zero-variable use of this method as "measuring the dependent variable twice, for the sake of security."

Lewin (1931) would have been surprised at the rational approach to classification. At the time of his critique of Aristotelian theorizing, the classification devices were more likely to be characteristics such as race, sex, age, or perhaps intelligence tests. Using such devices, the behaviors to be expected are not necessarily given within the categorizing device. The kind of consistency that he addressed was consistency among behaviors within a category, not consistency between a verbal description of a behavior and enactment of the behavior.

Perhaps one way of addressing the Nicholls et al. critique is to return to the state of affairs as it was at the time of Lewin (1931), and rework the zero-variable theories, in such a way that the classification device does not contain a seemingly redundant description of the behaviors to be expected. Instead of the usual modern, rational scale, one would substitute race, body type, gender, nationality, age, or some other nonverbal index, in order to divide people into categories (see Willerman, 1979). The primary difficulty with these seemingly antiquated methods is that the territory— the reach of one's system—cannot be well specified through such crude and undifferentiated classification criteria. That is, when the theorist brings age or race to the fore as a classification device, it is not immediately apparent what the behavioral domain is. But the rational scale construction method allows an easy and ready specification of the behavioral territory. Such a system resolves all ambiguity and also lends itself better to a unique name, thus guaranteeing the individuality of the contribution.

One of the curious aspects of the zero-variable approach and its dependence on the self-report of behavioral tendencies is that the theorist needs a good deal of faith in the respondent's introspective powers. For each of 20, 30, 40, or more behavioral instances, respondents are asked to indicate how much or how strongly they show the behavior (in general). The zero-variable theory assumes that the self-report will be consistent with the overall picture: the various behaviors must hang together positively, the reports of those behaviors must hang together positively, and verbal self-report must relate positively to the actual behavioral tendency. But this leaves the entire psychology of consistency out of the picture.

Neglecting the Psychology of Consistency

In a critique of S.L. Bem's (1974) androgyny concept, Pedhazur and Tetenbaum (1979) charged that such a system is nothing more than a simplified consistency theory. Subjects report how they would behave and then their behaviors are measured. The theorist, having no faith in "higher" psychological dynamics, remains entirely on the level of the behavioral outcome of psychological processes that are, in fact, neither assessed nor even acknowledged.

But consistency is a psychological process in its own right. Even if we neglect the psychological antecedents of subjects' verbal reports on the scales, a considerable amount of psychology can be brought to bear on consistency between report of behavioral tendencies and actual behaviors. One approach (Willerman, Turner & Peterson, 1976) asks subjects to state the most extreme behavior they can imagine, rather than their usual level of behaving. A statement of the most extreme imaginable instance appears to have more predictive power.

Another technique, developed by Fazio and Zanna (1978, 1982), assumes that subjects' self-reports need to be anchored in behavioral instances for the reports to be valid. Fazio and Zanna have developed a number of techniques for raising the salience of relevant behaviors, just before subjects give their self-reports. The result of such techniques is quite reliably an increment in the correlation between self-report and subsequent behavior. Still another approach, which has consistency theory thinking at its base, assumes that subjects will draw their self-reports and behaviors into coordination with one another primarily under conditions of self-focused attention. Numerous studies (see Gibbons, 1983, and Wicklund, 1982, for summaries) show that self-focused attention results in (1) respondents' bringing their behaviors into line with reported attitudes or values, and also (2) respondents' bringing their self-reports of behaviors into line with usual behavioral tendencies.

In short, one can draw on a variety of approaches, even theoretical statements, in the effort to increase the correspondence between what subjects say about themselves and how they actually act or perform. But here again the critique and prognoses of Lewin (1931) are to the point.

Denial of Psychological Consistency Processes

The Aristotelian model of theory-building was seen by Lewin as a statement about the fixed essence of the human. Once the person was assigned to a category, all elements (behaviors) within the category were assumed to correlate highly with the others quite automatically. If the essence of the individual was "spiteful" (two-year-olds), then all varieties of spitefulness would be shown. Other than category membership, the Aristotelian theorist saw no possibility for psychological forces acting on the individual to increase or decrease consistency among different varieties of spitefulness.

Our current Aristotelian models remain true to Lewin's characterization, some fifty to sixty years later. It is interesting, in examining the correlations reported in the preceding "external validity" research, that none of the investigators views the leap from verbal report of behavior to related (i.e., "external") behavior as a psychological leap. The correspondence is assumed to be automatic, inherent in the organism's ascribed essence, given that the organism is in the "average" situation. No single investigator raises the issue of whether certain psychological forces might eventually reduce that correlation to 0, or raise it to .99, or turn it into a negative correlation.[1] To do so would entail acknowledging the workings of psychological forces *outside* the particular zero-variable system. That such forces are never incorporated into research stemming from zero-variable theories signifies that the particular scale in question does have the

Aristotelian flavor that Lewin described. The functioning of the organism, at least within a certain area of complex human activity, is totally reduced to the classification instrument.

Increasing Consistency within the Zero-Variable Mode of Thinking

Throwing Out Inconsistent People

Without heed to psychological factors stemming from the organisms' perspective, the Aristotelian style of theorizing can be implemented to try to produce a tighter consistency within the categories. How does one go about this? For one, simply select out the people whose "nature" it is to be consistent, and disregard the others. Such an effort by Bem and Allen (1974) has been made famous. Respondents were asked to indicate how consistent they generally were within certain behavioral areas, then their actual consistency within those same areas was observed. Two classes were formed: individuals who claimed to be consistent across time or situations, and those who admitted to less consistency. Perhaps not surprisingly, those who claimed to be consistent showed more consistency. For instance, consistency on the friendliness dimension, between self-report and behavioral friendliness, was .61 for the "consistent" group and .06 for the inconsistent group. The conclusion of this study? Bem and Allen (1974) note that such a procedure should be a boon for personologists who are interested in increasing the magnitude of their "consistency coefficients"; when inconsistent people are expelled, correlations climb in the positive direction.

Averaging Across "Situations"

In characterizing the manner in which the Aristotelian theory develops laws about behavior, Lewin (1931) notes, "It is evident that no more is demanded of a law than a behavioral average. The law thus applies to an 'average situation.' It is forgotten that there just is no such thing as an 'average situation' any more than an average child" (p. 172). Thus the situation, rather than being viewed as an aspect of the individual's momentary psychological condition, is relegated to the status of a nuisance factor, which can only interfere with the operation of the essence of the organism. It becomes important, therefore, to be sure that one is dealing with an "average situation" when applying an Aristotelian principle.

Epstein's (1979) solution to the basic inconsistency problem reflects Lewin's characterization quite accurately: "People obviously do not manifest response dispositions independent of the setting. That is why it is usually necessary to cancel out situational effects, including subtle background effects that often go unrecognized, by averaging over occasions to demonstrate stability in behavior" (p. 1122). What is the empirical solution? Epstein proceeds to sample respondents' behaviors and self-reports of behaviors over a period of several days, finding that averaging these measures produces an overall heightened consistency. For instance, reports of one's heart rate over a twelve-day period appear to correlate with objectively assessed heart rate more than does a one-day sample of self-reported heart rate. In Epstein's view, this averaging over situations or time results in the ironing out of various situational influences that would otherwise contribute noise to the measure. But his method remains just as Aristotelian in character as the Bem and Allen (1974) solution: No matter which solution we elect to pursue, the psychological workings of the individual are progressively disregarded, or suppressed. With one solution the uncooperative (basically inconsistent) people are eliminated from the analysis; with the second solution the idiosyncrasies associated with individual cases of behavior are ironed out. The one effort thus improves the functioning of the eternal category by denying entry to uncooperative respondents; the other approach denies idiosyncratic, situation-specific actions. Neither of them refers to any psychological variables.

Neglecting the "Weirdo"

Another method of increasing consistency is to focus on the "normal" population. Similar to Lewin's (1931) formulation of the problem, the theorist stresses that the person-characterization and scale apply to *most* of the people, or to *most Americans*, or to *western peoples*, or something of the kind. These kinds of statements are seldom a regular part of the modern zero-variable theorizing, but the theorist has the possibility of referring to such notions on the grounds that a conservative statement is better; that is, it is safer to confine one's theoretical statements to a *known* group of people. An example comes from S.L. Bem (1974). In deciding which traits to include in the portraits of the "masculine" and "feminine" persons, the trait lists were generated in the context of such questions as "In American society, how desirable is it for a man to be truthful?" (Bem, 1974). If judges evaluated truthfulness as something that men in the United States should have, then truthfulness went into the masculinity scale.

Various zero-variable theorists' attempts to increase the tightness, or inner consistency, of their theories have been even more explicit than the effort by S.L. Bem. Indeed, these theory-tightening or category-shrinking efforts can well be regarded as part of the theorist's effort to build the theory further. But we will return to this theme in Chapter 12.

The next chapter develops the present theme a step further, and is based on the thesis that the zero-variable effort is bound up with the zero-variable theorist's striving for control. It is not sufficient to note simply the consistencies associated with one's categories; an overriding concern with the *power* of those categories is a frequent accompaniment.

Note

1. Depending on the psychological assumptions underlying a self-report scale, one should not be surprised at the emergence of negative correlations between a scale score and certain behavioral outcomes that would normally appear to "flow logically" from the responses to the items. For example, scale answers may well reflect a compensatory effort among individuals whose identities or egos have been threatened (see Wicklund & Gollwitzer, 1982). A related instance comes from cognitive dissonance theory (Festinger, 1957). People whose attitudes are relatively extreme, in a given direction, are particularly likely to shift far *away* from the position following the induction of dissonance (Cohen, Terry, & Jones, 1959). In other words, a marked *in*consistency in repeated responding to the same instrument is sometimes the best possible evidence for a theory.

9
Frequency, Power, and Accounting for All of the Variance

There are several ways for an observer, scientist, or other individual to control behavior. The one route, emphasized by Lewin (1931) under the rubric of Galilean thinking, is to investigate or examine the multiplicity of perspectives offered by the individual being studied, drawing on information about perceptions, motives, needs, chronic orientations, and so forth in trying to predict (and thereby explain) the individual case. Thus, to get a handle on the individual case, the observer should draw on pertinent aspects of theoretical wisdom and establish the combination of forces that influences the person at any given moment.

A good case in point is Festinger's (1954) social comparison theory. Even though the theory is frequently applied as an account of why people try to influence others, one cannot say that there are "classes" of individuals, some of whom have a strong need to influence and others whose need is slight. Rather, constellations of factors must be brought together simultaneously and applied to the individual case: the person's momentary need to gain clarity about a given opinion or ability, the momentary access to relevant, comparable others, the centrality/extremity of the person's opinion or ability relative to the others, and also the possibilities for cessation of comparison. Each time the person does something, such as exert influence on others or cease comparison by leaving the group, the system of psychological forces changes. In short, the Galilean mode of analysis does not allow the person to remain a static entity, *always* oriented toward Behavior X, nor does the subjective situation remain constant, *always* guiding the person toward Behavior X.

Frequency as Power

The Aristotelian mode of thought, as embodied in the modern zero-variable theory, adopts an entirely different strategy. Given that the background perspective and thus psychological variables are neglected, the only manner in which the investigator explains respondents' behavior is through the historically defined category (Lewin, 1931). "Historically defined" means that some facet of the respondent's previous existence, such as previous behavior (in this case questionnaire behavior), is taken as the criterion of category membership. But then what happens? The essence that is acquired through category membership becomes the sole force guiding behavior, and the investigator can only hope that the category-appropriate behaviors will be emitted *frequently*, regularly, or consistently. If we were to transform Festinger's social comparison theory into a zero-variable model, we would have to find an empirical way of distinguishing between "high social comparison need" and "low social comparison need" individuals.[1] Further, we would have to indicate the exact properties of each category, such as "high need people frequently try to influence others; low need people do this much less frequently." Behavior then becomes determined solely by this everlasting need.

Quite analogously, the concept of drives, for example, the hunger drive or the maternal instinct, is nothing more than the abstract selection of the features common to a group of acts that are of relatively frequent occurrence. This abstraction is set up as the essential reality of the behavior and is then in turn used to explain the frequent occurrence of the instinctive behavior . . . .(Lewin, 1931, p. 153)

For the psychologist who wants power in explaining, the result of the zero-variable formulation is a self-defeating one. Even though the theorist's purpose is to show that the category-pertinent behaviors are frequent (i.e., regular), the refusal to allow psychological forces into the explanatory system means that one's own system is necessarily weak. All possible explanatory factors and devices other than one's own categories are excluded, thus driving the theorist into the cul de sac of aiming to explain *all* behavior within the designated territory by means of a single dichotomy. And since this is impossible, a certain frustration should manifest itself as a by-product of zero-variable theorizing.

We should then be able to witness symptoms of the frustration within the language of the zero-variable theory. For one, the zero-variable manuscript should manifest an overriding concern with *power, proportion of variance explained*, the *constancy* of the effects, and the like. The zero-variable theorist, trying to explain tremendous areas of complex human behavior, simply cannot do it—the frustrations are objectively evident in the minimal sizes of the correlations between the scales and the "external validity" behaviors. The correlations indicate that the theorist can account for about 10 percent of the variation in the behaviors being examined. Thus 90 percent of what respondents do belongs to "alien" systems of forces. But are the irritations with this lack-of-power issue in fact manifested? Let's look at a few examples.

A Social Comparison Phenomenon: "My Own Scale Is More Powerful"

Given that the relationship between category membership and "external validity" criteria is generally minimal, the zero-variable theorist is obligated to find some *comparative* route to claiming power for the theory. A seemingly direct, though surprisingly infrequent, manner of doing this is to compare the power of one's own categories with that of competing categories. For example, Paulhus and Martin (1988), in representing the "functional flexibility" category system, begin by referring to Bem's (1974) androgyny as a competing notion of flexibility. The next step involves correlating each scale (i.e., their own and also Bem's scale, now called "flexibility") with a certain criterion, such as external ratings of subjects' flexibility. Admirably, Paulhus and Martin were able to prove that the correlation for their own scale was a bold .44, while that for the competitor was a mere .12.

Avoidance of these kinds of social comparisons seems to be more conspicuous in zero-variable reports than does the kind of exercise conducted by Paulhus and Martin (1988). The route more generally taken is characteristically that of showing relationships between one's scale and some external behavior or person-quality, but systematically avoiding the issue of whether someone else's scale might also predict that behavior. Potential problems, such as discovering that one's own system is not the most powerful, are solved by a policy of isolation, but only at the stage of predicting behavior. It is notable that the theorist is always interested in comparing category systems at the *scale* level—that is, discriminance analysis—but when the issue is the power of prediction, all comparison is suddenly dropped.

Social Comparison Again: "Individual Differences Are Stronger than Situations"

A theme that accompanies the zero-variable approach is the attempt to defend the power, or even existence, of chronic behavioral tendencies. A systematic Galilean analysis of the human would automatically regard this kind of defensiveness as meaningless, in that it is apparent that the person's entire perspective must be considered in a systematic analysis. Allport (1937), Cattell (1966), Crowne and Marlowe (1960), Lewin (1926, 1931), and Murray (1938) have had no problem with this kind of thinking. However, if psychologists think only on the level of the immediately observable, without constructs, then these kinds of "situation-versus-individual difference" battles become likely.

For example, a frequently cited article by Epstein (1979) attempts to prove that categories, defined through questionnaire responses, have a kind of constant, everlasting influence on behaviors. The language of his article is decidedly antipsychological, referring only to empirical events. Although the reference throughout is to *personality variables*, the reader would be wrong in supposing that Epstein's use of the term personality implies anything related to a psychological construct. He equates the term with observables. Attempting to rescue his "personality" concept from various attacks, which have charged that correlations between scale scores and behaviors are weak, Epstein adopts a defensive stand, then finds data that point to intraindividual consistency; and along the route, he tries to show that situations are not so influencial after all. Some short excerpts follow.

In citing a longitudinal study by Block (1977), Epstein makes it clear that stability coefficients involving personality and behavior can easily attain such levels as .70, meaning that certain behavioral dispositions tend to remain constant over long intervals. He then demonstrates within his own research that the predictability of a classification device is greater if the investigator takes the sum of numerous behavioral instances as the criterion. In explaining why the usual questionnaire–behavior correlations are so low, Epstein refers to the influence of the situation, but as a "noise" factor: "People obviously do not manifest response dispositions independent of the setting. That is why it is usually necessary to cancel out situational effects . . . by averaging over occasions to demonstrate stability in behavior" (Epstein, 1979, p. 1122). He then observes that one cannot really expect all behavioral dispositions to be manifested in all situations. Thus, "The fact that people read in a library and swim in a swimming pool does not establish that there is no generality . . . in either swimming or in reading behavior" (p. 1122). Then, noting that a global, cross-situations approach is needed to show intraperson consistency (what he calls "personality"), he concludes, "Given an adequate sample of occasions, however, response dispositions will out" (p. 1123) ("Will *win* out" was no doubt intended.)

If the reader has any doubt about the intent of the last quote, a further passage will clear up all ambiguity. Epstein explains that the prediction of individual behavior "with reasonable accuracy" (i.e., power) requires correlations in the vicinity of .80 or .90. And indeed, by examining individuals' *average* behavior over numerous instances, Epstein was able to obtain such lofty correlations.[2] Thus, it is obvious that the situation may be neglected: if the chronic behavioral tendency of the person accounts for 81 percent of the variance, the situation obviously must be relegated to an inferior status. At best, it could then account for only 19 percent of subjects' behaviors.

This situation-versus-individual-difference battle, waged necessarily on the level of empirical events, was continued in grand form in 1983 by Funder and Ozer. Once again recoiling at the charge that the "personality coefficient" is generally only .30 or .40,[3] Funder and Ozer set out to demonstrate that dispositional effects are just as potent as situational effects. How do they go about this? They select four "situational" studies on the basis of "their prominence in the literature of social psychology" (p. 108). Reducing each of these investigations (e.g., Darley & Batson, 1973; Festinger & Carlsmith, 1959) to a correlation coefficient, they show that the "situational" effects are not all that overwhelming, producing effects of only .36, .39, and so forth. They conclude that "the effects on behavior of several of the most prominent situational factors in social psychology seem to average slightly less than .40" (p. 110). It then turns out that dispositions, as well as situations, are important, even if they do not account for very much variance. Indeed, "It seems that there is no simple direct relation between size and importance of effects" (p. 111). If this is so, one wonders what all the commotion is about. And why were these particular four studies (situational variables) selected for examination rather than more explosive situational variables, such as sunshine and temperature? (see Cunningham, 1979, who reports correlations of .60 and .75 between sun, temperature, and reported mood.)

Are these kinds of exercises indeed a reflection of social comparison processes? The answer is easy to come by if we look at just two features of the Funder and Ozer comparisons. First, rather than examining the "average situation" in psychology, whatever that might be, they selected prominent, highly visible "situations." Second, they took care to be sure that the criterion correlation involving individual differences was placed at the level of .40, thus guaranteeing that individual differences account for *at least* as much variance as does the usual, prominent situational variable. This level of .40 is reputed to have come from an article by Nisbett (1980), but his meaning has been distorted. According to Nisbett, the characteristic correlation involving individual differences is in the range of .10 to .15.

In short, the Funder and Ozer exercise takes place independent of any considerations of constructs or psychological variables, and reduces the field to a level of strength of empirical events, which are selected in a seemingly capricious manner.

Concreteness in Aristotelian Thinking: Lewin's Critique

The concreteness, or positivistic nature, of these situation-versus-disposition controversies has not gone entirely without criticism. Block and Block (1981) refer to the problem inherent in psychology's "expressing a view of personality as no more than a bundle of unconnected dispositions, a set of differing probabilities to respond in different ways without regard for the specific environment context operative for the perceiving and responding individual" (p. 85). Indeed, Block and Block recommend the acknowledgment of psychological constructs—perceptions, motivations, and other psychological conditions—exactly the components that are seldom present systematically in situation-versus-disposition controversies.

In a still more direct commentary on these kinds of undertakings, Moos (1968) observes that the old question of situation versus individual differences is a pseudoproblem. The interests of the investigator and the character of the individual differences or situations that are chosen for study determine which side of this false dichotomy will dominate.

If we look carefully at Lewin (1931), we begin to gain some understanding of the importance of such situation-versus-disposition controversies for the zero-variable theory. The Lewin observation works in this way: The Aristotelian category does not acknowledge an inner, psychological life. Variables pertinent to cognizing, motivation, and the like are excluded totally. If the person is classified as optimistic, then a high frequency of optimistic manifestations must prevail; one has no other predictions, and no means of making a differentiated prediction. The investigator cannot say that the classifying instrument has operationalized optimism "weakly" or "strongly," since the act of categorizing is an all-or-nothing process: either the category member is an all-out optimist or not.

From that starting point, it then becomes important to apply the theory in normal, or *average*, situations (Lewin), particularly situations in which the list of behavioral tendencies is most likely to be observed. The frequency, as well as the strength, of the observed behavioral outcomes is what the theorist hopes to show, and the *average* situation, containing no rough corners or "abnormal" qualities, allows the categorized individual's essence to blossom in full form. It is perhaps no accident that zero-variable theorists, particularly the active situation-fighters (e.g., Epstein, 1979), place great emphasis on the undeniable practical significance of the categories in question. This orientation to the practical importance of the behaviors and the averageness of the situation is, in Lewin's words, "a requirement which, if transferred to physics, would mean that it would be incorrect to study hydrodynamics in the laboratory; one must rather investigate the largest rivers in the world" (p. 158). Given that the significance of the zero-variable theory lies totally in its potency, as applied to the average situation (as in Epstein's averaging-across-the-situation approach), it follows directly from our competition hypothesis that the theorist should be interested in making sure that alien concepts are not applicable in those same "average" situations. Thus, the investigator examines other efforts to account for complex behavior, sometimes even efforts that have a strong theoretical base, reduces those efforts to particular "situations," and then asks whether the situation or one's own category is stronger.

What does this look like in concrete terms? In the exercise reported by Funder and Ozer (1983), the "situation" abstracted out of the Festinger and Carlsmith (1959) experiment was the variable of payment; that is, some subjects were payed more than others. Similarly, the number of bystanders present became the "situation," as abstracted from the Darley and Latané (1968) research. The question then became, "How potent is the situation '$20.00'?" or "How potent is the presence of X number of bystanders compared to the situation composed of no bystanders?"

Lewin would have described this kind of business as the reduction of the person to a geographically based category. That is, for the purpose of the analysis, the respondents' essence becomes no more than their association with $20 or with two bystanders. Once the psychological constructs underlying these manipulatons are disregarded, it is then necessary, within the Aristotelian mode of thinking, to be concerned about the strength and reliability of such categories. A sensible question would then be, "Does Category X, based on a certain scale, or on race or gender, account for more behavior than a category based on $20.00 payment, or one based on the presence of two other people?"

Although Lewin (1931) could not have foreseen the issues associated with social comparison and competition among zero-variable category owners, we can now see the direction in which the modern zero-variable theory must develop. Given that the empirically defined category is the only component of the theory, the theorist is obligated to show that it is potent. When this cannot be done in an absolute manner, for instance, by inflating one's correlations through eliminating inconsistent subjects (see Bem & Allen, 1974), then the potency is attested to by showing the *relative* power of the system. That these kinds of exercises are necessarily selective and capricious is well illustrated by the pitting of a monetary category ($20.00 payment) against a scale-based category (Funder & Ozer, 1983). The so-called situationist, functioning in this same positivistic, concrete mode, would seek out situations with undeniable strength, comparing them against a selection of disposition categories that does not appear to relate very well to certain behaviors. To be sure, there is an alternative to this fruitless activity, but the alternative requires that we depart from the Aristotelian mode of theorizing. This brings us to the next section.

The Functioning of Constructs: Frequency and Power Are Not the Criteria

Construct versus Empirical Category

Reactance (Brehm, 1966; Brehm & Brehm, 1981) is not an empirical event, even if a peripheralist, objectivist, positivist, mechanist, elementarist (see Murray, 1938), or single-operationalist (see Campbell & Fiske, 1959) would try to reduce it to one. Reactance is a construct, and the sense of a construct was given quite clearly in the writings of Cronbach and Meehl (1955) and others, as discussed in Chapter 7. Reactance is postulated as an internal condition of the human, a motivated condition, in which the reactance-laden person strives toward reestablishing specific behavioral freedoms. The multifacetedness of this striving is, of course, observable; assessing or inducing reactance is also an empirical matter. All of these empirical endeavors have the character of operationalizations: the operationalization is said to set off, instigate, assess, or measure facets of the reactance construct.

What would be the shape and form of reactance as reduced to an empirical category? Lewin (1931) suggests two possibilities for this Aristotelian endeavor. The human is reduced to an essence *historically* (e.g., high-reactant people versus low-reactant people) or *geographically* (either a person is in a "reactance situation" or is not in a "reactance situation"). Taking the historical approach, reactance is reduced to the visible, tangible contents of the questionnaire used to define the reactant person. Taking the geographical technique as a starting point, reactance is translated into the person's association with a "reactance-situation." With such an Aristotelian theory, the operationalization of the construct is no longer an issue, because there is no construct. There is only a person, whose totality is reactant or not reactant. It makes no sense to speak of "operationalization of a type of person," since the person is already a concrete entity. What are the implications of these Galilean/Aristotelian differences for the kinds of research questions that are asked?

Taking the Galilean approach, the investigator begins with a certain confidence in the lawfulness of relations among reactance-relevant variables. For example, the interworking of (1) a respondent's degree of expectation of freedom and (2) subsequent constraints on behavioral possibilities is a central aspect. Thus, a setting is arranged in which respondents expect more (or less) freedom within a given choice context; constraints are then placed on the options. For instance, a woman might expect freedom in selecting a date from several males; another woman might expect less freedom (Wicklund & Ogden, in Wicklund, 1974, pp. 113–115). As the second step, the behavioral possibilities are reduced, through sudden absence of one of the males, for instance. Reactance (the construct) is thus operationalized—through the combination of a high expectation about one's own freedom and the curtailment of that freedom (sudden absence of a choice alternative). The hypothesized outcome, an orientation toward reestablishing the threatened freedom, is then measured.

How strong and how frequent is the reactance response? Such questions are completely irrelevant to the theoretical enterprise. The investigator's purpose is to reach inside the respondent's perspective, to get a handle on the hypothesized relationship between expectations of freedom and curtailment of choice. The frequency with which the subjects would "normally" show such reactions, or the absolute strength of such reactions, is of no concern to the investigator. There are two reasons for this:

1. The theorist's or investigator's attention is on the lawfulness of the postulated principles, not on the frequency or strength of the reaction. Thus,

whether the freedom-seeking reaction carries over into the next day or is stronger than the freedom-seeking efforts in "everyday life" is not in the forefront of the investigator's attention.

2. The size and regularity of the behaviors depend on the potency with which the construct is operationalized. "Expectations of freedom," as a theoretical construct, is not reducible to "choices in the grocery store" or "choices among life occupations." The expectation can be induced, thus operationalized, across a spectrum of potency levels. The important point is that the investigator who is interested in the functioning of the *construct* does not care about its degree of power. Given that an infinite number of operationalizations is possible, one can magnify the functioning of the construct accordingly.

Therefore, the Aristotelian institutions of sampling across "average situations," seeing that the effects are stable across some arbitrary time/space dimension and that the investigation corresponds to "real life" conditions, may all be neglected, quite correctly, within the Galilean method of scientific psychology. The criteria of success, for the theorist, have nothing to do with power and frequency.

If we take the frequency and power criteria away from the Aristotelian school and ask the zero-variable theory to adopt the criteria of the Galilean system (perhaps as a kind of role-playing exercise for the zero-variable theorist), what would happen? The theorist would have to shift attention to the systematic relationships between variables that operationalize the construct. But let's try to search for the variables. By distorting the terminology, the zero-variable theorist might say, "my scale operationalizes the construct androgyny," that is, "my variable is the dimension androgynous/not-androgynous." Good! And now the second step: How does this so-called variable relate to other theoretical variables? The answer here is, "it relates to the behaviors that are predicted from the theory." What behaviors? Those used to define the categories in the first place.

One begins to understand why frequency, consistency, and power are the only reasonable criteria of success for the zero-variable system. The theorist has no other direction in which to turn.

Notes

1. It is not difficult to conceive of a scale that would be created for such categorizing: Cacioppo and Petty's need for cognition scale could be taken as a model. One would list behavioral instances that, in the investigator's mind, constitute "comparing" behaviors, all of this predicated on the implicit assumption that such needs show no flux.

2. Although the methods used by Epstein are not of central importance here, the reader should be cautioned: Epstein's subjects were commissioned to keep track of their feelings, phone calls, social contacts, stomachaches, and so on every day, for a period of fourteen days. The monumental consistencies he reports are

based on these cumulative self-reports. For instance, as the days wore on, subjects tended to report always having the same number of social contacts. Thus, whether there were any important consistencies across actual objective behaviors remains an open question.

3. Funder and Ozer (1983) refer to Nisbett (1980) as maintaining that correlations between dispositional variables and measures of "experimental behavior" (their formulation) are seldom above .40. They then proceed in the course of their article to treat the .40 value as a standard against which to compare "prominent social psychological" findings involving experimental variables. The reasoning is difficult to follow, particularly since Nisbett's (1980) summary refers to correlations that are characteristically within the .10 to .15 range, given that dispositional measures are correlated with behaviors phenotypically different from the measuring instrument used to assess the disposition. In short, the statistical standard for comparison that should have been selected by Funder and Ozer is the correlation of .10 to .15. As this chapter tries to demonstrate, the relative sizes of these "person effects" and "situation effects" are not pertinent to the present discussion. The point here is that such comparisons make sense only when a positivistic psychology replaces a psychology of constructs.

10
Suppressing Alternative Explanations

The completed zero-variable theory, as we have witnessed the course of its formualtion, is an egocentric product. The respondent's background perspective is shoved aside as the theorist attempts, through discriminance analysis, to win a unique place in the field of verbal description of complex human behavior. A further element now enters the antiintegrative picture: nowhere in the zero-variable literature is the concept *alternative explanation* taken seriously. In other words, the perspectives of other theories are neglected, not just the perspectives of the respondents. Before we develop this theme, it is useful to take a quick look at the usual character of the alternative explanation; what does it mean in psychological research and what are its consequences?

An Example: Cognitive Dissonance Theory

The development of investigations of cognitive dissonance theory (Festinger, 1957) has been accompanied by a sharp eye toward constructs that would serve as alternative explanations of the results. One of the earliest published, relatively thoroughgoing attempts at an alternative explanation was by Rosenberg (1965), who charged that the characteristic dissonance-arousing paradigm creates "evaluation apprehension." According to Rosenberg, this is a kind of refusal to bribed by the experimenter, particularly by large monetary reimbursement. Thus, the construct "evaluation apprehension" replaces the construct "cognitive dissonance." Rosenberg allows that evaluation apprehension leads directly to resistance to attitude change, since the experimenter, offering high monetary incentives, presumably favors such attitude change. The direction of the thinking is clear: The Festinger and Carlsmith (1959) payment of twenty dollars brought about evaluation apprehension and resistance to change, relative to the subjects who were payed only one dollar. This is, then, a clearly formulated alternative explanation.

Linder, Cooper, and Jones (1967) acknowledged this alternative explanation, then considered the issue from the perspectives of both theories. Given that dissonance theory includes the variable *volition* (Brehm & Cohen, 1962), Linder et al. conducted a further experiment in which some of the subjects wrote a counterattitudinal essay under conditions of relatively free choice, while other subjects were constrained in writing their essays. The idea is that an open misrepresentation of one's own opinion will create cognitive dissonance, but only if the counterattitudinal act is undertaken of one's free will. To be sure, they obtained the expected results. Important here is that the construct "evaluation apprehension" carries no such free will variable, which means that the total pattern of the results in the Linder et al. experiment cannot be reinterpreted as an "evaluation apprehension" phenomenon.[1]

We should note once again that this kind of consideration, whereby one's attention is drawn back and forth between different explanations, is possible only as long as one is dealing with a psychological construct. If the original Festinger (1957) statement had simply been, "Hypocritical behavior results in attitude change," no one would have quarreled with the statement on the level of an alternative explanation. The reason is that a mere statement of an empirical relationship constitutes no explanation, thus does not call *alternative* explanations into the picture.

The Alternative Explanation Within the Zero-Variable Theory: What Can It Look Like?

In the previous chapter we saw that the zero-variable theory has no operationalizations; there is no construct to be tapped into. Accordingly, one may not charge the zero-variable theory with refusal to consider *alternative* psychological constructs, since the core of any zero-variable system is, itself, not a psychological construct. The list of behaviors in the theory's scale operationalizes nothing; it is just a list of behaviors.

Nonetheless, there are possibilities for the zero-variable theory to break out of total egocentrism, in the sense of acknowledging others' approaches. And the direction for such breaking out is clear enough: each zero-variable theory lays claim to a certain behavioral territory, a territory that is characterized within the scale and which is also claimed in the course of doing "external validity" exercises. Each theory is set on accounting for a maximum number of the frequent behaviors within its chosen domain, thus coming out of egocentrism implies a recognition that others can also account for behaviors within that territory.

Again, the reader might keep in mind that the acknowledging of others' theories, within the zero-variable exercise, cannot mean comparing one's own psychological variables with the other's variables, as in the cognitive dissonance example. Nor can it mean comparing two constructs. There are no constructs or variables to be compared. At this point, we shall have a look at our central examples, to examine the extent to which theoretical perspectives other than one's own are acknowledged. The overriding question is, "To what degree are others allowed in one's own territory?"

On the Level of the Categorizing Device

The question of whether others intrude on one's own territory is expressed in very different forms. For instance, Carver and Scheier (1981) refer to the possibility of "alternative explanations" for the effects of chronic self-consciousness; to rule out one such alternative explantion, they carry out a discriminant validity test against the social desirability scale. Similarly, Cacioppo and Petty (1982), in finding no correlation between their own scale and social desirability, conclude that social desirability does not *bias* responses to their scale. Paulhus and Martin (1988), also fighting against the social desirability scale's possible intrusion, checked to see whether their scale was "contaminated" by social desirability. S.L. Bem (1974) performs the same kind of analysis, using her own social desirability scale, and concludes that androgyny is something different from a "general tendency" to respond in socially desirable ways. And Snyder's (1987) classification system is not "simply" the need for approval (i.e., social desirability).

Thus, practically every theorist shows a strong concern that social desirability might have a claim to the behavioral territory, and such claims are irradicated on the level of scales, by proving no overlap between two measuring devices. All of this is on the verbal level; what do we see when we move to the level of more overt behaviors, the behaviors that are referred to in "external validity"? (see Chapter 8).

On the Level of Nonquestionnaire Behavior

Seldom is a correlation between the theorist's scale and a behavior examined through the perspective of a competing categorizing device with an interest in discovering whether that other device accounts for the behavior at least as well. A rare instance is Snyder's (1987) examination of certain behaviors in light of the Crowne and Marlowe (1964) social desirability scale. Snyder begins with the finding he documented earlier, that high self-monitoring is associated with skill and willingness in communicating feelings. Then comes the crucial issue: does social desirability also predict such behaviors? Snyder's (1987) answer is that people with high need for approval are *less* able than those with lower need for approval to communicate feelings (p. 25). This analysis, then, evidently allows the self-monitoring scale free reign in the territory of "communicating feelings."

But let's follow this reasoning one step further. If the social desirability tendency and the self-monitoring categories really do not overlap in territory claimed, then this should apply to all territories that fall under the rubric of one or the other system. As it turns out, the authors of the social desirability scale have conducted numerous investigations. Let's see what correlates with social desirability, as reported in Crowne (1979).

The Domain of Social Desirability

Looking first just at other measures that overlap with social desirability, we see that the MMPI *Lie* scale correlates highly with the Crowne–Marlowe scale (.54). An interesting fact. The self-monitoring scale refers explicitly to the willingness to lie, that is, the theory is clearly meant to apply to lying behavior. In order to clarify which system has a greater right to the territory of "lying," it would be sensible to look at the self-monitoring–lying relationship. It may well be that this part of self-monitoring's territory is already taken.

How about the tendency to create a positive impression within a social context? Crown and Marlowe (1964) report a study of implied demand for conformity to the wishes of an experimenter. True to their expectations, subjects high in social desirability were more inclined to communicate to the experimenter that the study was enjoyable and of high scientific importance, and that they would like to participate in more such experiments. But this happens to be the territory of the self-monitoring scale, and of the Fenigstein et al. (1975) public self-consciousness scale. Suddenly we have at least three scales fighting to explain the same behavioral domain. How do we decide who wins, or who is entitled to account for such experimenter-friendly reactions? Given the criterion of validity for a zero-variable theory (i.e., strength of relationship), the only reasonable step is to find out which of these three competitors accounts for *more* of the behavior in question. Thus, according to correct zero-variable reasoning, they should be tested for relative strength, in the same manner as Snyder's (1987) route to the dismissal of social desirability as an account of expressiveness.[2]

The social desirability findings cumulate: there is also a strong positive relationship between social desirability and inhibition of aggression (Fishman, 1965). Again, we see a potential realm of application for self-monitoring and public self-consciousness; the self-monitoring and self-conscious individual should be prone to withhold aggression to please the other. A comparative test between these systems is needed to see which one generates the strongest correlations.

Our question here is a simple one. Given that the criterion of a zero-variable theory is the strength of the scale-behavior relation, why hasn't the comparison between self-monitoring and social desirability been carried out on the behavioral level? For instance, can the self-monitoring scale "predict" conformity behavior exactly as well as social desirability does, and if it cannot, then—on the basis of zero-variable thinking —self-monitoring must be regarded as the less appropriate account of conformity.

A still more interesting case involves a potential contest between self-monitoring theory and category of public self-consciousness. In one empirical study using this self-consciousness scale, Solomon and Schopler (1982) examined the extent to which respondents attended to current fashions in clothing; high public self-consciousness types attended more to current clothing modes. Slightly later in this same historical period, Snyder and De-Bono (1985) report a positive relationship between self-monitoring and interest in the image of consumer products. Given that the effects being measured (interest in modes, image, or modern attire) are similar for the two efforts, the way is opened for a mutual challenge: which zero-variable theory accounts for the most variance in the world of mode (style orientation)? The presence of a high correlation between the *scales* in question (.45, in Cheek, 1982) should have stimulated the authors to address the issue of which theory should rightly claim modes and styles. But such direct comparisons have never been made.

As a kind of validity index for their flexibility measure, Paulhus and Martin (1988) obtained information on their subjects' skills in dealing with social situations, adjusting to new social situations, appearing likable, and acting appropriately in social settings. This is a perfect validity index for public self-consciousness (see Fenigstein, 1979) and also for self-monitoring. A three-way comparison should thus ensue, to establish which of the three can account for more of the variance—that is, show the most power—on the Paulhus and Martin validity index. The loser would then be advised to retreat from the territory of "skill in social situations, appearing likable, acting appropriately."

A Two-Fold Egocentrism

The Perspective of the Respondent

A cornerstone of the zero-variable approach is the disregard of the respondent's background perspective. The rise and fall of perceptions, motivations, behavioral readinesses, and developmental antecedents of category membership are all suppressed and supplanted through the category-defined essence. This means that any interpretation of the behavior (arguing, complex explaining, lying) that refers to such inner states, or to the changeableness of the subject, must be swept aside. There is no way, from the standpoint of the zero-variable mode of thinking, to acknowledge those processes.

Even when subjects themselves offer complex explanations for their own behaviors, as White and Younger (1988) have so amply demonstrated, the zero-variable theory would not be capable of recognizing those accounts as alternative explanations of what is going on. Rather, the zero-variable explanation more resembles the *observer* perspective, also assessed in White and Younger, which reduces the observed person to a static entity—a package of traits and physical characteristics (see also Sande, Goethals & Radloff, 1988; Wicklund & Braun, 1987).

If the zero-variable development refuses to allow the explanations that respondents give of their own behavior, then a Galilean account of behavior—which emphasizes the several factors bearing on the person—must also be denied. In essence, the self-observer as an explainer is differentiated, makes reference to changeable psychological states, and considers factors that bear on change. The zero-variable manuscript gives no heed to the existence of these kinds of explanations, neither to respondents' accounts of their own behavior nor to Galilean accounts of those same behaviors.

The Perspective of the Other Zero-Variable Theories

Even if the language of mutually competing zero-variable theories is on the same level (i.e., almost all of them deal with behavior lists as the starting point), there is no recognition that one's competitor also addresses the territory of interest. We have seen sufficient examples. This refusal to compare, on the behavioral level, seems remarkably blatant when we consider the overlap between theories in scale content. If two scales both address conforming behaviors, independence, and gullibility, shouldn't the authors be interested in knowing whether the competing scales also show a close correspondence to actual behaviors? For example, numerous items of both the need for cognition scale (Cacioppo & Petty) and the attributional complexity scale (Fletcher et al.) refer to respondents' orientation toward an intellectual climate.[3]

As one external validity check, Fletcher et al. (1986) gave subjects the option of selecting simple or complex explanations for a given event, and true to expectation, the high scorers (complex subjects) chose the complex explanation. It would have been an easy matter, however, to check whether the earlier formulated need-for-cognition scale (Cacioppo & Petty, 1982) would have predicted just as well. And if it had, this acknowledgment of the Cacioppo and Petty perspective would have led Fletcher et al. to question their territorial claims.

This illustration of refusal to look at another perspective represents a widespread phenomenon, which has nearly no exceptions. The reason for the phenomenon has presumably to do with the theorist's avoidance of unfavorable comparisons, which in turn could spell a loss of territory. Should it turn out that our competitor can explain 30 percent of the variance in intellectual functioning but that our own scale accounts for only 25 percent, there is a loss of relative power. Is there an alternative to fall back on then, to shore up one's own theory? The only remaining possibility is to point to other segments of one's territory, hoping that the predictive power of the scale is higher than that of alien categories. But this is a dangerous game, whose outcome is unclear, and it can result only in the eternal search for territory segments that bring one's own power back into a favorable light. Thus, we should expect no efforts to acknowledge other accounts, and certainly no efforts toward integration, among the zero-variable formulations.

Notes

1. Results paralleling those of Linder et al. have also been reported by Frey and Irle (1972), Holmes and Strickland (1970), and Sherman (1970).
2. The distinguishing mark of the Crowne and Marlowe contribution is that they have a *theory*, in which other psychological concepts play a role, particularly avoidance and fear (see Crowne, 1979, p. 182). Furthermore, the developmental side of the approval motive is considered and researched. One cannot say that the theoretical side of the approval motive depicts the human as a static, either–or entity.
3. A sample of items from the Cacioppo and Petty scale makes this point evident:

   No. 4: "I would prefer a task that is intellectual, difficult, and important to one that is somewhat important but does not require much thought."
   No. 13: "I prefer just to let things happen rather than try to understand why they turned out that way."
   No. 23: "I would rather do something that requires little thought than something that is sure to challenge my thinking abilities" (scored negatively).

11
Categories: The Good and the Bad

Lewin (1931) observed that the Aristotelian version of theorizing was inevitably fraught with value judgments, or value-laden concepts. For instance, the dividing up of people into higher and lower IQs cannot be separated from value judgments, as witnessed in the way the IQ concept has been treated through history (Kamin, 1974). And in the older "socio-logical" theories of racial differences in artistic or economic potential (discussed in Sorokin, 1928), one sees that the "Aryan peoples" are supposed to be more valuable to the universe than the "Alpine" peoples.

The Psychology of Person Perception

The zero-variable theory treats the human as an intact unity that displays a certain essence. If everyone can be said to possess or not possess that essence, it is a short leap to society's evaluation of the usefulness or accep-tability of that essence. And depending on which segment of society, or which historical phase examines the dichotomy, the value judgments will change. The psychology of person perception (Hastorf, Schneider, & Polefka, 1972) allows us to conclude that a person, as a constant unity, is invariably evaluated, particularly insofar as the person has relevance for the perceiver. This is such a taken-for-granted, matter-of-fact phenomenon that the concept of evaluation has long since been built into the concept of attitude (McDougall, 1908).

On the other hand, an examination of the respondent's perspective, in the context of a theory with variables, is not necessarily accompanied by an evaluative attitude toward the person as a unit. Let's examine why this is, in the context of Zajonc's (1965) social facilitation theory. First, Zajonc does not regard the individual respondent as a unit. Instead, the potential behaviors of the subject, and the habit strengths underlying them, are ex-amined with respect to a given setting. For example, a particular habit, such as standing up when the national anthem is played, might be very strongly trained in, or less strongly trained. Second, the amount of arousal induced in the person is the other critical element of the theory. To the extent that arousal (drive) is high, owing for instance to the presence of an audience, the habits with greater strength tend to appear and suppress behaviors that are less well trained.

What could evaluation look like within such a context? No doubt, the observer could make evaluative statements about the character of each habit, but there is a qualitative difference to the zero-variable theory. Rather than summarily evaluating the *entire person* as modern, socially tuned, and so forth, the evaluation must be oriented toward individual habits. In short, a theory with variables, which allows the respondent to change, eliminates the possibility of relegating the entire person to a positive or negative category.

The necessity of a prior person-categorization for a person-evaluation has already been demonstrated by Fiske and Pavelchak (1986). Only to the degree that a person fits firmly into a comprehensive category is a strong evaluative response to the person possible.

At this point we will look at our five central examples, plus a few more, to see the form that evaluation takes in the context of the zero-variable theory.

Argumentativeness

Along with the person-characterization of the argumentative type, Infante and Rancer (1982) ascribe some qualities to the "high" type that are ostensibly valued, at least within an academic culture: the person finds arguing to be an intellectual challenge, experiences excitement and invigoration on such occasions, and has self-confidence. The poor "anti" type, being low on the scale, is stuck in the position of not seeing arguing as intellectually challenging, as not experiencing excitement and invigoration (but instead *fear*), and has little self-confidence in debating settings. The overall portrait of the positive category is of an individual who is highly communicative, good at debating, and generally, a highly valued member of a modern, educated society. The person who scores low does not fit well in a modern, educated, verbal caste. Some further distinguishing characteristics support this overall value-laden dichotomy: the "highs" also earn better grades in school. Interestingly, they are also more politically conservative. Whether this last point fits the overall, positive picture depends on the subsegment of educated, verbal society to which one belongs.

In case the reader has noted that argumentativeness might also be objectionable in certain circles, surfacing as obnoxiousness or aggressive attacking of others, Infante and Rancer (1982) reassure us that this is not so. The argumentative person would certainly not attack or humiliate another to inflict psychological injury (p. 74). Thus, the argumentative type is not only socially skilled, communicative, and self-confident, but is also a basically nice person.

Eliminating the Extremes

Infante and Rancer are also attentive to the possibility that extreme scorers might not be such socially valued people; for instance, it is suggested that the extremely high scorer might be an "incessant arguer" whose behavior would "impair interpersonal relations" (p. 80). The authors do not like the idea that such undesirables might be part of the favored category, and they propose the following solution: "If research reveals that extreme ARG_{gt} scores [high argumentative people] are symptomatic of difficulties in interpersonal relations, it should be possible to develop techniques for moving people from the extreme regions of the trait argumentativeness distribution" (p. 80). The direction of the thinking is straightforward: the zero-variable theorist does not like the idea that socially unwelcome behaviors might stem from the favored category.

Self-Monitoring

The "high" category was originally the one favored by Snyder (1974). The high self-monitor was the socially skilled, flexible, perceptive, managing type who left a good impression in social situations. The low type was a socially inept, sometimes naive, uninteresting type, who always behaves the same, no matter what the situation. Here is a clear similarity to the socially competent/socially incompetent pictures drawn later by Infante and Rancer.

Somewhat later Snyder (1982) upgraded the valuation of low self-monitoring people. The cross-situational consistency of such types, and the consistency between verbal statements and self-descriptions, was placed in a laudatory light. The grayness and social ineptness of the "low" type was, as of 1982, underplayed. A step later Snyder (1987) devoted considerable discussion to the evaluation of the two types, stressing the idea that both are good people: "Nevertheless, to characterize the low self-monitoring sense of self as principled is not to confer on it any special ethical or moral status. . . . there are no reasons to regard either self-monitoring type as inherently better or worse than the other" (1987, p. 51).

Androgyny

The positive evaluation of a type of person is seldom more pronounced than in S.L. Bem's definition of androgyny. The components of the masculine and feminine scales are traits that are (or at least were) highly socially desirable among modern academics. The criterion used to select traits for the masculine or feminine scales was as follows: "because the BSRI was founded on a conception of the sex-typed person as someone who has internalized society's sex-typed standards of desirable behavior for men and women, the personality characteristics were selected as masculine or feminine on the basis of sex-typed social desirability. . ." (1974, p. 155). Since the androgynous person is a combination of masculine and feminine leanings, one must conclude that the androgynous person is portrayed in Bem's definition as the best possible sort of person (at least in the eyes of the judges who decided which traits were masculine-desirable and which were feminine-desirable). The further value-laden aspect is in Bem's assumption that "rigid sex-role differentiation has already outlived its utility" and it is hoped that "the androgynous person will come to define a more human standard of psychological health" (p. 162).

Thus, the hero in this theory, the androgynous person, is modern, sensitive to others, psychologically healthy, and self-confident—an image of the ideal person that runs through all three of the conceptions discussed so far.

Attributional Complexity

The attributional complexity theory (Fletcher et al., 1986) moves away from the idealized portrait of the modern, socially skilled, communicative, self-confident person and in the direction of intelligence. The valuational character of the person high in attributional complexity is spelled out in considerable detail by Fletcher et al.; here we touch on just a few facets of this gleaming characterization. Among other identifying characteristics, the "highs" are said to be intrinsically motivated to understand human behavior, are more curious about others' behavior, prefer complex explanations, tend to infer causality from the individual's past, and think about the "underlying processes" involved in causal attribution.

Is this a picture of a socially desired type? It is reminiscent of the Piagetian youth who has just evidenced prowess in hypothetico-deductive reasoning, who plays with concepts, draws complex inferences, and tries out hypotheses. Thus, the "highs" of Fletcher et al. are cognitively mature, alert, and have a good deal of analytical intelligence. They are no doubt valued by the academic community.

The portrait of the "lows" is not spelled out explicitly, but if we do this, the evaluative character of the dichotomy immediately shines through. This is a person who is unmotivated to understand others' behavior, prefers simple explanations, does not like to think about underlying processes, and is not too bright. People in this category are cognitively immature in a Piagetian sense. It is clear that much of educated society does not like such people.

Need for Cognition

Cacioppo and Petty's (1982) concept differentiates between people who "engage in and enjoy thinking" and those who are less inclined in this direction. The valuational aspects are obvious.

The Self-Knower

Another typology that has become popular among zero-variable formulations is the self-knowing individual. For instance, in Buss's (1980)
characterization of the "private" self-consciousness category, the person
who scores high on the ten-item "private" scale is said to be more introspective and to have more accurate insight into the inner workings of the
self, particularly with respect to potential for behaving. Markus (1983),
regarding the person with a strong self-schema as an individual with high
self-knowledge in a given area, has built the self-knower category into a
highly laudatory group. The person who scores extreme on a given dimension and finds that dimension to be important is thus a member of the
self-knower group and possesses a certain "expertise" and "competence"
in the area of interest (e.g., extraversion; masculinity/femininity). The self-
knower can thus make faster decisions in the area of self-knowledge and
has more experience and is more competent in that area, compared to the
non-self-knower.

Functional Flexibility

The superiority of the favored category is seldom more emphasized than
in the Paulhus and Martin (1988) treatment of the flexible person: "Functionally flexible persons possess a great many interpersonal capabilities:
They have a large repertoire of social behaviors and can deploy these behaviors in the situations they deem appropriate" (p. 99). Flexible persons
are viewed as being psychologically healthy, having high self-esteem, and
knowing what behaviors will bring them the best gains in the long run. One
can only pity the respondents who lie below the median on the flexibility
measure.

Three European Races

The idea that there are superior groupings of people, whether one
focuses on social relations or on intellectual and creative matters, has a
direct counterpart in the writings of de Lapouge (1896; see Sorokin, 1928,
p. 234). For instance, the highest category in de Lapouge's system, the
Aryan race, is viewed as taking great risks and thereby achieving incom-
parable successes: "Progress is his most intense need" (Sorokin, p. 235).
There is nothing the Aryan type does not dare to think or desire, and
desire for him means realizing it at once. His religion is Protestant, i.e., the
Aryan stands for "progress." In comparison, the groups Homo Alpinus
and Mediterranean are treated as sub-standard within de Lapouge's
system.

De Lapouge props up the validity of his theory by claiming that the Nordic, or Aryan, race has been responsible for all important cultural achievements, and further, that education cannot correct the inherent differences in these three racial groups.[1]

Even though the de Lapouge categories antedated our other examples by roughly eighty years, a continuous theme is present in the evaluation criteria. The hero for de Lapouge is the active, progressive, modern person—the individualist—and the talented and successful. Specific comparisons with our contemporary examples are not necessary: the overriding similarity is that the modern, accomplished person rises to the top. The activities of people in this category then become the standards by which others are evaluated.

Explaining What Is Good

The Lewinian (1931) charge that Aristotelian thinking is bound up with evaluative thinking is apparent enough from our examples. But a more interesting point, one that could not have been recognized in Lewin's time, is the manner in which the modern zero-variable theory focuses on the accounting for "good" behavior. The moment that something unwanted creeps into the desired category, the theorist undertakes changes to ensure that everything is all right, that is, that nothing societally unwanted remains in the category. ("Societal" refers to the norms of the theorist's own reference groups.)

A striking example comes in a radical revision of S.L. Bem's theory by Bem et al. (1976). In the original theory (1974) androgyny was defined in terms of the absolute difference between tendency-to-masculinity and tendency-to-femininity. If the respondent scored zero on both the m and f scales, the difference score was of course zero, indicating a very high level of androgyny—a balance between the two tendencies. If the respondent scored at the highest possible level on both the m and f scales (let's say 100), then the androgyny level was also defined as high.

But then came a discovery: the people whose androgyny came into being through the combination of low m and low f scores showed singularly low self-esteem. This was not acceptable to the hero conception that had been built around the androgynous person. As a result, the low–low group was redefined as "nondifferentiated," thus as no longer androgynous.

Problems can also arise for the zero-variable theory's hero portrait when the behaviors stemming from high scorers have shades of antisocial meaning. This happens quite easily in self-monitoring research. For example, the alleged social skills and flexibility of the high self-monitor can be shown to relate to more frequent changes of friends and partners (Snyder, 1987). One way of looking at this (Snyder, 1987) is through the generous view of the high self-monitor as a functionally thinking, careful planner. For instance, it is noted that high self-monitors seem to assign their friends to special situations—a friend for parties, a friend for studies, and so forth. In comparison, low self-monitors content themselves with long-lasting and less-differentiated friendships. Examining the results from another perspective, one concludes that the high self-monitor is unfaithful and handles his friends and acquaintances in a malicious, instrumental manner. This kind of problem is handled within the self-monitoring school by means of carefully chosen euphemisms and attention given to the possible positive shades of meaning. For instance, instead of "unreliable," the high self-monitor is seen as being flexible and adaptable in interpersonal matters (Snyder, 1987).

Staking Claim to a Positive Territory

In each of the theoretical characterizations we examined in Chapter 4, the author's focus was on the positive side of the dichotomy. For the most part, the reader gains the impression that very little attention is given to the "low" category and that the theorist is seldom interested in explaining the disvalued person's behaviors. Obviously it is necessary to see what the negative person actually does, when conducting external validity research with behavioral criteria, but the reader's attention is invariably guided to the socially adroit, communicative, nonneurotic, intelligent, clever functioning of the positive type. This focus is reflected in the theoretical "system's" name: in none of our examples does the title refer to the undesired category—for example, "undifferentiated" (S.L. Bem), "attributionally simple" (Fletcher et al.), or "without need for cognition" (Cacioppo & Petty). Rather, the theory is named for the hero in the system—the complex, socially skilled, modern individual.

This forces us to reconsider what might be meant by laying claim to a behavioral territory. It now begins to look as if our previous conception was not quite on the mark. That conception portrayed the modern theorist as scanning a large field of complex social behavior and picking out behavioral elements that seemed to have some commonality and which would lend themselves to unique packaging under a heretofore nonexistent label. That is not quite right. Instead, the theorist—at least among those we have examined—scans to find various behavioral tendencies that would fit into a unified *hero* portrait, a portrait that the theorist's reference group would welcome as a seemingly superior type. This is, then, a portrait of a person with whom the theorist would not mind being associated. In the present cases we are dealing with heroes in social relations (Bem; Infante & Rancer; Snyder) and, on the other hand, heroes in the cognitive–intellectual realm (Cacioppo & Petty; Flechter et al.).

If we were to translate this kind of pursuit to other theoretical realms, we would have to assume that, for instance, Schachter's (1964) theory of emotions would treat only positive affect. Similarly, theories of attitude change would concentrate on attitude change in a socially useful, laudable direction. This is, of course, impossible in the case of a psychological theory that is composed of constructs and psychological variables. If we concentrate our research efforts on variations in a psychological state, then the behavioral consequences are a matter decided by what the variables produce, not by the theorist's desire to represent instances of "positive" human functioning.

But what is the reason for this overemphasis on the hero figure, the type with a pleasant mix of culturally valued qualities? This tendency seems to be a systematic accompaniment of the theorist's decision to develop a zero-variable theory, and the focus on a hero figure may even antedate the development of one's own zero-variable theory. Certain directions of societal change should have to do with the potential theorist's focusing on a societal ideal as the center of the theoretical work. One would guess that the salience of women's emancipation was not entirely irrelevant to the development of androgyny classifications. And Fletcher's attributionally complex person was a seemingly timely effort, coming directly in the aftermath of social psychology's long-lived preoccupation with relatively "simple" attributional processes. The Fletcher attributors are capable of something more sophisticated than is dictated by attribution theories. On the other hand, one cannot really argue that the argumentativeness scale was the result of a cultural wave of concern with debating or arguing, and in general, it would not be prudent to say that all such theories are the immediate outgrowth of a societal emphasis on particular human talents.

But there is still another possibility—a simpler alternative: "Would you rather associate yourself with a positive, or a negative person?" Theorists who are interested in making a unique contribution, who want their names on a theory, have a certain investment in seeing that the entity for which they stand is a culturally prized one. The zero-variable theorist prefers not to point to the category of the disfunctional, the non-respected, or the neurotic. At least, this appears to be the case for the relatively recent zero-variable systems.

Association with a Category Replaces Perspective-Taking

In a sense, the psychologist builds a bond to the person who is being studied. In the ideal case, as illustrated in the first two chapters, this bond involves the psychologist's openness to the multitude of perspectives offered by the respondent. The subject's historical background, mental states, motives, habits, dispositions, perceptions, and changeableness are followed and described by the theorist. But what occurs when this perspective-taking approach to theory-building is rejected?

A bond remains in any case, but in this case the bond must be between a *person-type* and the theorist, *not* between the complexities of the perspective and the theorist. That is, given that the Aristotelian mode of theorizing reduces each respondent to a static, concrete entity, the psychologist's association with that entity automatically acquires a highly evaluative character, in that each category carries a highly evaluative loading. Given that a bond necessarily exists, a loose derivation from Tesser's (1986) thinking about social comparison leads us to the notion that theorists would try to associate themselves with a group (category) that carries a positive image.

We can formulate this idea on a still more concrete level. The zero-variable theory entails two lists of behaviors, or two categories—the one list consisting of elements that spell out something favorable within the theorist's culture. Assuming that the self-esteem maintenance processes described by Tesser (1980; 1986) are applicable to the behavior of psychological theorists, it stands to reason that theorists would build a bridge between themselves and the culturally valued behaviors—modernity, communicativeness, flexibility, alertness. Since the theorist's connection to the respondent's perspectives has been eliminated, the only remaining bridge is to the concrete behaviors of the respondents, and working from the Tesser notion, associations to the positive elements will be emphasized.

Accordingly, it does not suffice simply to note that theorizing by means of categories is associated with evaluative thinking vis á vis one's subjects or patients. The evaluation is of a particular kind, based in the theorists' emphasis on the cultural superiority of their favored categories, while the less favored category is downplayed. For the most part, the characterizations of the two categories read as though the theorist would be quite happy if the inferior category were to slip silently away; one sees little interest in "explaining" the behaviors of the unfavored group.

Note

1. Sorokin (1928) levels a thorough criticism against such racist schools of thought, focusing particularly on the fallibility of the criteria that had been used to divide Europeans into the three racial groupings. In addition, Sorokin points to evidence that contradicts the common assumption that fair-haired people make their way to the top of the social heap. For instance, "Of 424 British men of genius, 71 were unpigmented (light), 99 were light medium, 54 were doubtful medium, 85 were dark medium, and 115 were dark fully" (p. 275).

12
Directions of Development for the Zero-Variable Theory

The major defining steps in the development of a zero-variable theory have been outlined in the previous chapters. But what next? Does development of the theory come to a halt with the demonstration of quasi-discriminance and external validity analyses, or can further steps be taken?

Subdividing the Categories

While the author of a zero-variable theory is seldom agreeable to the re-working or redefining of the original categories, it occasionally happens that a subdivision takes place within a particular zero-variable territory. Lewin (1931) had foreseen this direction of development when he suggested that the progression of Aristotelian thought moves in the direction of ever-finer, increasingly narrower categories, thereby ensuring an enhanced consistency among the symptoms (behaviors) within any given category. What does such subdivision look like in the modern zero-variable theory?

A classic example is found in the androgyny theory, consisting of a change introduced two years after the system was first published (Bem et al., 1976). Originally Bem (1974) dealt with three categories: masculine, feminine, and androgynous. This third and all-important category consisted simply of people whose m and f scores were about euqal, no matter whether high m and f, or relatively low m and f. Then the bomb dropped (Bem et al., 1976): The low/low group evidenced a lower self-esteem than was warranted by the notion that androgynous people manifest only "positive" characteristics.[1] The solution was simple and congruent with Lewin's prognosis: to tighten the internal consistency of the system, the low-feminine/low-masculine people were relegated to the category "undifferentiated," while the high/highs remained in the preferred category "androgyny."

In principle, similar kinds of subdividing can be carried out with any such system, the criterion being that internal consistency within categories should increase. An interesting, somewhat complex case in point is the Fenigstein, Scheier, and Buss (1975) double self-consciousness concept of "private" and "public" self-consciousness. Each type of self-consciousness has its own scale, thus each respondent can be placed into a high or a low public category as well as into a high or a low private category.[2]

Miller, Murphy and Buss (1981) redoubled this effort, differentiating between *body* self-consciousness—private as well as public body self-consciousness—and the ordinary, more general self-consciousness that was originally addressed. Logically this gives us eight possible categories. While it remains to be seen whether there are payoffs in terms of better within-category consistency, the eight-cell system obviously is reason for optimism. One hopes that the predictive power of a classification system will be stronger the further it breaks categories down into minicomponents. This kind of development is reminiscent of the actuarial approach taken by an automobile insurance company, whereby driving record, alcohol use, age, sex, and education are all entered into the probability-of-accident (i.e., "risk") term. It is simply assumed that a system with many subcategories will predict more successfully than one with only two categories. This is, then, the source of optimism behind this direction in theory development.

Gender is also a very likely basis for the further carving-up of one's category system. Fletcher et al. (1986) note that women "are more interested in people than men are—that they are keener naive psychologists" (p. 877). In short, if we know that a respondent belongs to the biological category *women*, we expect her to be higher in attributional complexity. Combining gender with the attributional complexity scale, we arrive at four logical categories, with "female-highs" and "male-lows" constituting the two extreme cases. Why was gender selected as the further classification criterion? No justification is given, aside from the previous quote. The empirical fact of the usefulness of another category is sufficient basis for introducing the category into the system.

The Fletcher et al. (1986) use of gender does not stand alone in the literature. Anderson and Thacker (1985), for instance, found it useful to combine the categorizing systems *gender* and self-monitoring. An analogous use of the gender variable, or occasionally the sex-role scale (see S.L. Bem), is found in a variety of other research, with the overriding justification for introducing gender (or genderlike categorization systems) being that it *makes a difference*. A quotation from Wolfe, Lennox, and Hudiburg (1983) illustrates the purpose of such combined categorizing systems: "When subgroups are defined by sex, analyses of reported alcohol use yield small but significant moderator effects: Women's use is more predictable from environmental variables, whereas men's use is more predictable from dispositional variables" (p. 1069). If such a conclusion is supposed to represent some broader conclusion about human nature, it is that men's behavior stems directly from some chronic "essence" (dispositional variables), whereas women's behavior can better be related to the environment. This leads us to another widespread option for categorizing people.

Geographical Classifications

Thus far we have focused exclusively on classification systems that Lewin (1931) termed "historically based," in the sense that they involve something out of the individual respondent's past. There is good reason for this focus. The modern zero-variable classification systems that attempt to account for complex social behavior have relied almost exclusively on the "rational" questionnaire approach to classifying the individual, thus little can be said about other types of systems, perhaps classification devices that stem from earlier periods. Some of these earlier classification systems were, of course, based on entirely different criteria, such as race, age, and biological gender. But the point here is that classification devices can also derive from the individual's environment (i.e., situation).

In the case of our five central examples, the historical aspect was the subjects' reports of their usual prior behavioral tendencies. Other historically based classifications can be made on the basis of age, gender, race, birth-order, and so forth. On the other hand, a *geographically* based classification criterion should serve the Aristotelian classification enterprise just as well. This means simply that the subject's essence is defined by environmental surroundings.

How does this work? The geographical basis for category-building brings us far afield from the rational method of questionnaire construction. For instance, within the geographical school of sociology, Ratzel (in Sorokin, 1928, p. 178) argues that states with large territories, simply because of their geographical greatness, tend toward expansionism, militarism, and optimism, whereas states with relatively small territories show more pessimism and lack energy. According to the reasoning, the energy level, optimism, and certain other qualities of individual citizens are defined by the geographical unit to which each citizen belongs. Murray (1938) calls such theorizing "physicalism"; the physical surroundings of people lead directly to certain reactions, and their background perspectives, motives, and perceptions are neglected.

Modern counterparts to the older sociological theories (i.e., the geographical and climatic theories) can still be found. Cunningham (1979), for example, has reported a number of relations between aspects of the weather and both helping behavior and mood. One simple finding among a sample of waitresses indicated a clear relationship between sunshine and self-reported mood—a correlation of .60. A still stronger effect was found for the relationship between temperature and mood (a correlation of .75).

Although the strength of these results is astonishing, the reader should not be led to think that there is anything psychological about these geographical–climatic explanations. The form of the explanation reads, "A person whose situation is defined as X is inclined to show Behavior Y." Conceptually there is little difference between this kind of theory and the theories based on historical criteria: "A person of race X, or who is above the median on Scale Z, will show Behavior Y." One sees no construct, no background perspective, and no psychological variables.

Combining Geography and History: Making the Zero-Variable Account Complex

The ostensible utility of geographical conditions has been seized upon by one branch of modern psychology, sometimes referred to as "the psychology of the *situation*." A striking example of the implementation of the situation is reported in Pervin (1981), where the possibilities for subcategorizing the essence of the human are taken to extreme.

In a project by Champagne (cited in Pervin, 1981), the central element was the *situation*. Each of twelve female subjects listed twenty situations that were representative in her current life. Then, for each of these twenty settings, the subject was asked to rate the likelihood of her exhibiting each of fourteen behaviors in that setting. For example, the subject would rate the likelihood of the behavior "smile a lot" in the situations "classroom," "football game," "on a date," "studying in the library," and so forth. One sees that a great deal of perseverance and tolerance was required of the respondents. All told, 280 likelihood ratings were required.

Here we see the potential of the idea of the "situation multiplied by the person." It does not suffice simply to classify people into categories of "friendly" or "not friendly"; instead, such person-categories must be qualified in terms of the situation in which they are shown. Using such a classification system, the elegant simplicity of our earlier five examples is lost; one cannot any longer argue that Disposition X will continually make itself known across all average situations. Rather, one's essence is defined by the combination of geography and behavioral disposition. This kind of system describes 280 separate, presumably reliable essences.

Champagne qualifies the system still further by asking each subject which of nine kinds of reinforcers would follow, given the occurrence of a particular behavior. We now have to subcategorize each of the 280 categories according to reinforcement type, requiring a total of 2520 judgments.

One can see that the introduction of subjects' reports about reinforcers into this multimatrix is an attempt to make sense of complex social behavior in terms of learning theory, but it is also apparent that the physical, concrete level is the one preferred for analysis. The theorist can only hope that subjects' retrospective reports have some bearing on their behaviors, as divided into this multitude of categories.

The use of situations, as in the Champagne approach, does not automatically render categories psychological. The 280-fold system just described asks subjects, for example, how friendly they would be in the classroom, how friendly at parties, and so forth. *Friendliness* is nothing more than a description of a behavioral tendency, and is on the same level as the descriptions among the scales of the five theories dealt with earlier. Similarly, situations such as *classroom* or *party* are nothing but physical characterizations. Thus, again, we have a complete absence of psychological variables. The Champagne system does not inform us as to the respondent's perceptions or motivations, and we are left in the dark as to *why* friendliness would be shown by Subject X in the classroom more than in the library. In other words, a zero-variable theory is just as feasible with 280 categories as it is with the usual minimal two categories.

Combining Geography and History: Reducing Theories to Categories

A novel manner of bringing a great many person-categories to bear on situations has been proposed in recent years by Bem and Funder (1978), Bem and Lord (1979), and Funder (1982). The starting point of the analysis is the selection of *situations* that have been implemented earlier, by other authors, to test theoretical notions. For example, one setting that Bem and Funder (1978) and Funder (1982) began with was the forced-compliance setting, in which subjects are requested to defend an opinion that is at variance with their own beliefs. This paradigm ("situation") was implemented earlier, on numerous occasions, to look at the variables stemming from cognitive dissonance theory (Festinger, 1957). Numerous studies have implemented the forced compliance paradigm to study the effects of such variables as the amount of discrepancy between the subject's overt opinion and prior opinion, the degree of justification offered for role-playing a discrepant opinion, and consequences of such role-playing (see Brehm & Cohen, 1962; Wicklund & Brehm, 1976).

The Bem and Funder (1978) approach begins with such paradigms, and then asks what type of person, within that particular setting, should show the expected reaction. In fact, the reasoning goes a bit further. Expert judges are first supposed to familiarize themselves with several theories (e.g., cognitive dissonance theory; self-perception theory, Bem, 1965) that might be applicable in such settings. Second, those judges are shown 100 traits (e.g., "negativistic"; "introspective") and asked to rate "the relevance of each of the 100 Q-sort items [traits] to the theoretical predictions of these theories. Each item was rated as positively relevant to the theory's prediction, negatively relevant, or irrelevant" (Funder, 1982, p. 104).

In turn, it was possible to examine the trait profile of each subject, and to predict how much attitude change the particular subject should show—all on the basis of whether that subject's traits were judged to fit more the "dissonance" personality, the "self perception" personality, or some other personality.[3]

The Theory is Eliminated

Although the justification for such procedures sounds elegant, in that the methods evidently allow comparisons of the strength of particular theories within a given setting, none of this research pays any heed to the contents of the theories involved. It is simply noted that a given situation is relevant for several theories, but the variables of those theories are not introduced systematically into the setting. And in place of the theoretical variables, certain "experts'" judgments about 100 traits are taken as the basis for knowing whether particular subjects are more (or less) inclined to behave in accord with cognitive dissonance theory or with other theories. Such a procedure takes the workings of the theory out of its network of variables, and redefines it in terms of observers' judgments about whether a given trait profile is suited for the experience of cognitive dissonance, self-perception, and so forth. Assuming that the procedure is successful, using the usual criterion of accounting for more variance (Funder, 1982, p. 106; see also Note 3), the authors do not indicate why their theoretically irrelevant use of traits is more on target than a theoretically relevant use. Completely neglected is an entire literature on the operationalization of dissonance theory variables through individual differences (Cohen, Terry & Jones, 1959; Glass & Wood, 1969). By no means can anyone argue that the Bem and Funder (1978) technique involves operationalizing a theory. Instead, the technique involves simply the observer's ("expert's") judgment about the "kind of person" who is "most likely" to experience dissonance.

How Many Situations; How Many Behavior Tendencies?

The number of situations psychology uses to test its concepts is seemingly unlimited, suggesting that the Bem and Funder technique would quickly lead to the problem associated with the Champagne project (see preceding text). Theoretical progress à la Bem and Funder would entail picking out the three or so most prominent settings used in testing each of twenty or so prominent theories, and then constructing a trait profile (from 100 traits) for each of those sixty combinations. Then, to discover how a given subject will behave, we need only consult the matrix to find (1) which setting is present, (2) which theory is being considered, and (3) what kind of profile is relevant. In the course of all this classification, the original constructs disappear; the pertinent variables and their operationalizations are shoved aside.

Bem and colleagues suggest that the raw material of the theory (i.e., the theoretical variables) is not enough for full understanding of the psychology of the subject. The theorist requires a bit of additional help from certain "experts," whose wisdom about the traits said to be appropriate to the theoretical process is greater than that of the theorist. The "expert" is presumably in the position of looking at the 100 Q-sort traits (intellectual, negativistic, irritable, submissive, power-oriented, anxious, etc.) and knowing that certain constellations of them are related to the "cognitive dissonance experience" in given situations while others are not.

Complexity Confused with the Background Perspective

The potential direction of development for the zero-variable theory is toward a finer mincing of categories. This further subdivision can be done with additional historical criteria (i.e., behavioral tendencies) or geographical criteria. Many observers would be inclined to judge such development as moving the "theory" in a more psychological direction, toward the actual complexity of respondents' true psychological worlds. But let's address this confusion.

If a psychologist takes the Galilean direction in analyzing the psychological background of behavior, then attention is given to events that have occurred earlier, in the respondent's personal past, and also to the psychological events that must be inferred—motives, perceptions, habits. The result of this route to psychologizing is the observation that certain sets of variables affect one another, that the interplay of these variables sets certain psychological conditions (i.e., perceptions, motivations) into play, and that these conditions then have a bearing on behavior. This kind of behind-the-scenes observation has been referred to as perspective-taking throughout the earlier chapters.

In the course of this approach to theorizing, the explainer obviously takes into account numerous geographical and historical elements, insofar as they are pertinent to the psychological condition being studied. But these historical and geographical elements are not simply picked out just because they exist. Rather, they are examined through their role in operationalizing psychological constructs.

We may return to Atkinson's (1957) theory of achievement motivation for an example. Persistence at certain tasks is often the behavior (dependent variable) of interest, and for theoretical reasons, certain facets of the subjects' backgrounds are considered at the outset. For instance, the relative strength of the dispositions "achievement motive" and "failure anxiety," and the probability of success, are regarded as belonging to subjects' perspectives—as steering their total approach/avoidance tendencies, and thus their persistence in the task.

Let's suppose that a hypothetical second group of researchers enters the scene and decides that Atkinson's system is not sufficiently differentiated. Subjects are further divided into age and gender, and their situations are divided into the categories of "work" and "leisure." These additional categories are shown to have a certain predictive value for the behavior *persistence at tasks*, thus it is concluded that achievement motivation theory is obligated to acknowledge the workings of these additional all-important elements. For the most part, the field of psychology would be agreeable to these additions, since one is inclined not to reject a more differentiated view.

Does this differentiated view have anything to do with Atkinson's original theorizing? Or, stated differently, does it have anything to do with the perspectives that Atkinson had traced in the course of constructing the theory? One is inclined to say "yes," but only because the categories sex, age, and leisure/work seem to be related to persistence. On the other hand, the psychologist who introduces these changes never answers either of the following questions:

1. How are age, sex, and leisure/work relevant to the psychological condition of the subject? Does "masculine" or "feminine" relate in some important manner to the arousal of achievement motivation? Is one race or another automatically predisposed to experience more achievement motivation? The "theoretical modification" never takes into account the perspective of the respondent. Rather, the modification consists simply of the statement that the original author's dependent variable is somehow affected by capriciously chosen categories.
2. In what way are the suggested categories (sex, etc.) to be integrated into the original theory? Is Atkinson, for example, now obligated to regard these categories as an integral part of achievement motivation theory? One sees that these kinds of modifications involve complete disregard of the *theorist's* perspective, and not just that of the respondents.

This direction of zero-variable-theory development, toward ever-finer distinctions among categories, brings us back to a theme covered earlier. The direction of development is set through the goal of the zero-variable theory, which is necessarily a *power* goal. Lacking variables, the only use to which we can put the zero-variable system is that of explaining variance, which means that the categories will be adjusted in any manner possible to squeeze out progressively more predictive power. Ultimately one reaches the absurdity symbolized so deftly by the Champagne (in Pervin, 1981) way of doing things: For every conceivable emission of behavior, within every conceivable geographical setting, a category must be made, all in the hope that the respondent's essences are stable enough to bring such a cross-tabulation to function predictively.

Notes

1. The low/low group proved to be unsatisfactory as "true" androgynous people in still further respects:

    . . . at least among men, they were also found to disclose less personal information about themselves to others; moreover, low-low scorers were found to be significantly less responsive to a baby kitten than high-high scorers; furthermore, in both the independence and the kitten studies, excluding the low-low scorers from consideration did serve to strengthen the original findings for both sexes. (Bem et al., 1976, p. 1023)

2. The concept *self-consciousness* was divided on the grounds that one needs both kinds of self-consciousness for purposes of prediction. Whether there can be two psychological forms of self-consciousness (i.e., self-focused attention) was not seen as a pertinent issue. To be sure, there is no basis for thinking that the "public" variety of self-consciousness has anything to do with the focus of attention on or away from the self (see Stephenson & Wicklund, 1983, 1984; Wicklund & Gollwitzer, 1987).

3. Interestingly, these investigations showed no evidence that the so-called experts could tap into the workings of cognitive dissonance through the 100 items in the trait list. The conclusion appears to be that cognitive dissonance is not relevant to its own paradigm, a conclusion that is remarkable in light of earlier evidence pointing to the motivational character of such forced-compliance paradigms, and also to the necessity of subjects' experiencing a cognitive discrepancy (see Cohen, Terry, & Jones, 1959; Pallak, Brock, & Kiesler, 1967; Waterman, 1969).

13
Is the General Direction of Theoretical Development Downhill?

The zero-variable theories touched on thus far have been regarded as set entities, as systems that have not yet been modified. On the other hand, one can regard a theory, no matter how Galilean or Aristotelian, as a step in a direction, as a member of a theory-chain, in which numerous theorists participate. Such a chain of theory-building takes place over years, possibly spanning cultural shifts, methodological developments, and generations. Such theorists as Harré and Secord (1972) and Kuhn (1962) have discussed these phenomena in theory-building as "paradigm shift" or "Old Paradigm versus. New Paradigm"; constellations of social factors would seem to play a stronger role in theoretical shift than does empirical evidence.

Chains of theoretical development may also be examined over a very short time interval, and our purpose in this chapter is to ask what happens to a theory once it falls out of the hands of its author. Does the next generation continue to treat it as a theory?

Murray (1938)

Let's see what Murray's aspirations were at the outset of his often-cited theoretical work: "Since psychology deals only with motion—processes occurring in time—none of its proper formulations can be static. They all must be dynamic in the larger meaning of the term" (p. 36). Among some of his primary propositions (pp. 38–49) one sees in Murray's thinking a view of the dynamic, multiply determined organism:

The organism is not an inert body that merely responds to external stimulation. Hence the psychologist must study and find a way of representing the changing "states" of the organism. . . . Since, at every moment, an organism is within an environment which largely determines its behaviour, and since the environment changes—sometimes with radical abruptness—the conduct of an individual cannot be formulated without a characterization of each confronting situation, physical and social. (p. 39)

Murray elaborated extensively, during the first seventy to eighty pages of his book, on the changing character of the organism, the waxing and waning of needs, conflicts, interacting patterns among needs, and the necessity of addressing the individual's subjective perception of the situation of its own needs. In this respect Murray was no less universal than Freud (1920), Lewin (1926), or Allport (1937).

But then what happened? Hilgard's (1987) analysis of the end result—the ultimate reception of Murray's (1938) book—reads as follows:

Henry A. Murray (1938) entered the field of human motivation by proposing a long list of human needs. The list was comprehensive, but not very systematic. . . . The reception of Murray's list in detail was never enthusiastic because his elements sounded too much like the earlier list of instincts, which indeed they reflected. . . . One of the needs that Murray stressed, the need for achievement, . . . became the mainstay of a long-continued research into achievement motivation initiated by David McClelland. . . (Hilgard, 1987, p. 364).

Hilgard goes on to note that Murray's other theoretical concepts, which were so central to the building of a dynamic theory of behavior, have been neglected. The primary elements that have remained, which have been influential in research and have played a role in further development of theory-building, are the "Murray needs." And how have these needs been used since then—primarily as Aristotelian categorizing devices, for example, "The person is basically high or low in 'succorance' or 'aggression.'"

All reference to the role of the press of the situation, to conflict among needs, to the rise and fall of specific needs or drives within the individual, has been shunted aside. Murray (1938) may have anticipated this disappointing development: "Positivists are usually disinclined to accept the concept of drive, because they cannot, as it were, get their hands on it. It seems like a vague, airy conception—perhaps a disguised emissary of theology and metaphysics" (p. 63).

Achievement Motivation

Taking one of the Murray-defined needs (achievement) as a starting point, McClelland and co-workers (1949, 1953) worked out an extensive theory. The developmental aspects of the achievement motive, its waxing and waning, and its influence on thinking and behavior were all drawn into the theoretical development. A highly systematic version of this notion was then developed by Atkinson (1957). According to the McClelland and Atkinson conceptions, the achievement-motivated individual was not *always* prepared to manifest the achievement motive. The time and place of achievement motivation peaks were said to depend on deprivation from achievement, cultural influences, other competing motives (see Murray), and concrete situations that set off achievement striving. These systems were very Galilean and, in fact, Atkinson (1964) gives a good deal of credit to Lewin's form of theorizing.

How has this thinking been developed further? Perhaps the most extreme form of "Aristotelianization" of the Atkinson and McClelland work owes to Mehrabian (1969), whose instrument asks respondents what they typically do. For example, one item confronts subjects with the hypothetical situation of having insufficient time to complete two projects, and then asks whether they would proceed to work on the more difficult, or the easier, of the two.

If we examine Mehrabian's enterprise in light of the accumulated Atkinson and McClelland research findings, it looks like Mehrabian has transformed earlier *dependent variables* directly into a rationally constructed scale. In turn, this means that research efforts within the context of this scale involve little more than measuring subjects' "chronic tendencies" (e.g., preference for difficulty) per paper-and-pencil, and then validating the scale by observing whether subjects show consistency between scale and overt behavior.

Rotter

Rotter's (1966, 1975) theoretical system may be regarded as an elaborate learning theory, in which the development of an individual's expectations regarding reinforcement is central. Crucial to the system is the analysis of the individual's background: One needs to know what sorts of contingencies or noncontingencies the individual has been confronted with in order to tap into the person's further expectations regarding control (as opposed to randomness) in further settings. These learned expectations can, within Rotter's system, also be *un*learned, or extinguished, when the reinforcement contingencies are no longer present.

Rotter's concept of learned expectations was highly differentiated. He referred to the individual's specific expectations, that is, expectations within particular settings, and also to generalized expectations. He assumed that expectations about reward contingencies generalize so highly that one can speak of a personality disposition. As a tool for tapping into the individual's generalized expectations regarding control (or contingency between one's own behavior and outcome), the Rotter team of Phares, James, Liverant, Crowne, and Seeman developed a rather simple scale, whose items tap into the person's beliefs about whether the world is controllable by individual efforts. In no way was Rotter's intention that this scale supplant his entire theoretical reasoning or render unnecessary further modes of inducing (or tapping into) the psychological condition of feeling of control.

How has the concept been developed? A good illustration comes from

Mirels (1970), who found that the Rotter IE scale can be factor-analyzed into at least two groupings. One group of items seems to refer to the subject's inclination to emphasize hard work (and not luck) as a determinant of outcomes. The other group of items appears to refer to beliefs about whether a citizen can influence world affairs.

In what sense do these kinds of procedures qualify as theory development? If we return to Rotter's original statement, we see simply that the IE set of items was intended as one possible operationalization of the individual's generalized feelings about control. Rotter would not have ruled out other operationalizations, nor would he have neglected the background factors that lead to such generalized feelings of control (or lack of control).

In a 1975 article on problems and misconceptions plaguing the internal/external control construct, Rotter points to the shallowness of some of the applications of his construct: "Without doubt, the most frequent conceptual problem on the part of a number of investigators is the failure to treat reinforcement value as a separate variable" (1975, p. 59). As further point, Rotter observes that researchers repeatedly try to find relationships between generalized expectancy (IE scale) and achievement behavior, and that such hypotheses become unreasonable insofar as a particular achievement situation is structured, familiar, and unambiguous.

If Rotter (1975) may be said to have a thoroughgoing complaint about the manner in which his theory has been implemented, it is that investigators have neglected the variables. Expectancy (which is not always handled correctly) is one such variable, the value of the reinforcement is another, and the character of the situation is still another. The situation is said to be pertinent to expectancies and to reinforcement values. In short, his reflective comments support the view that the development of his theory has been in the direction of a one-sided emphasis on the omnipotence of the scale.

In countless articles that have appeared since 1966, the IE scale has been incorporated, with the overriding assumption that the *highs*—people with a stronger sense of personal control—are less likely to give up, are more hopeful, show more persistence, are more resistant to intrusions, are more successful, are more task-oriented, and so forth (see Gore & Rotter, 1963; Lefcourt, Lewis & Silverman, 1968; Rotter & Mulry, 1965; Strickland, 1965). The "further development" of the theory takes the form of always dividing respondents into "internals" and "externals," and then showing the superior performance, rationality, or endurance of the internals.[1] The 0-variable character of this development is exactly as clear as it was with achievement motivation. The original theorist's relatively differentiated analysis of the background of the individual respondent, including the analysis of individual expectations in specific settings or changes in the sense of control expectations, is replaced by a dichotomy—the constant "highs" versus the constant "lows."

Learned Helplessness

In the original theoretical approach of Overmier and Seligman (1967) and Hiroto and Seligman (1975), helplessness was regarded as a psychological condition that entailed an overgeneralized reaction to repeated noncontingencies within a given setting. The earlier research demonstrated these generalized effects rather directly, with the subject's feeling of control being a very important factor in the generalized effects. For instance, in research by Glass and Singer (1972), severe noise caused later performance decrements (i.e., the generalized effects) only if the noise constituted an *un*controllable element in the person's environment.

Shortly after its inception, this general line of thinking was elaborated by Wortman and Brehm (1975). The theoretical statement was expanded to include performance *increments*. The critical variables were (1) expectation of control, (2) importance of the control, and (3) amount of threat to or degree of elimination of control. Based on research by Roth and Kubal (1975), Wortman and Brehm (1975) indicated how one would go about testing this elaborated model of helplessness. The intriguing and highly dynamic aspect of this elaborated theory was the idea that constraints on the individual's freedom, security, or possibility of behaving, could generate either of two opposing reactions: helplesness and related effects, as shown by Hiroto and Seligman, or performance *increments* (Roth and Kubal). Depending on the constellation of background factors, including the intensity of the helplessness training, the importance of the behavioral area, and the subject's prior expectations about control, the Wortman and Brehm theory made precise predictions about the form of reaction that should occur. What has happened since the introduction of this seemingly comprehensive model? The demise of the theory has taken at least two steps.

The first step was an "attributional" rewriting of the learned helplessness notion (Abramson, Seligman, & Teasdale, 1978). Helplessness was said to ensue if the respondent experienced uncontrollable outcomes and also made a so-called global attribution. This development is worth noting because (1) the model allows no way of knowing when or why a person would make a global attribution, and (2) the performance *in*crements and other pertinent variables stipulated by Wortman and Brehm are neglected. The theory, in its Abramson et al. form, is now reduced to the idea that helplessness effects owe to global attributions, even when the forces behind "globality" are not known to the theorist.

The second step, initiated by Peterson, Semmel, von Baeyer, Abramson, Metalsky, and Seligman (1982), reduces the helplessness undertaking to a simple scale, and the behaviors of interest are reduced to depressive symptoms. The idea behind the scale is to assess subjects' chronic tendencies toward certain attributional styles; the people focused on as respondents are those who manifest internal, stable, and global attributions for unwanted outcomes. As Peterson, Villanova, and Raps note, three years later (1985), the idea of a relationship between what they call attributional style and depressive symptoms has become a frequently researched area; they refer to sixty-one published studies.

In the meanwhile the variables that were pertinent at the time of Glass and Singer (1972), Hiroto and Seligman (1975), and Wortman and Brehm (1975) have vanished. Along with those variables, the manifold outcomes of the construct helplessness have also been brushed aside. The primary remnant of the original formulation is the empirical relationship between a type of person (one with a tendency to accept blame for unwanted outcomes) and certain symptoms labeled "depression."

Summary

These examples are found in numerous domains in psychology. As soon as a theorist makes a statement about the psychological condition of the human, involving the convergence of several factors on the growth and demise of that psychological condition, further development of the theory reduces the psychological condition to a tangible, fixed device—based on the respondent's history or geography—that categorizes the person. Thus, the development of theories across short time spans, across methodological developments, or over generations, shows a decidedly unidirectional tendency: the construct and thus the manifold perspectives of the individual are rapidly shunted aside in favor of concrete categorizing devices. The criterion of the "developed" theory is then how well the investigator can predict specific instances of behavior.

Such a development cannot be traced directly to a general decline in the readiness of psychologists to think psychologically.[2] No matter when in recent history a broad theoretical statement about psychological processes has been proposed, the researchers/theorists who immediately follow undo the theory in the direction of a zero-variable concretization.

What brings these short-term simplifications about? Does it suffice to postulate a general human tendency to reduce psychology to empirical categories? In the following, several psychological theses are put forward to explain the "simplicity-drift" or "positivism-drift" in psychological conceptions about the human.

Control, Commitment, and Competition

One way to examine this issue, drawing on the concepts of Chapter 2, is to consider the situation of an aspiring theorist or researcher who attempts to do *something active* with a previously formulated theory. At a minimum this would entail using the theory to predict, and thus to gain control over concrete individuals' behavior. To the extent that this orientation toward control of behavior is strong, the symptoms we have examined in Chapter 1 should appear: simplification of the theoretical system and the tendency to view the objects to be controlled as having permanent, predictable characteristics. In contrast with the nonactive *reader* or *observer* of the theory, the person who uses the theory in an active way should be expected to move the interpretation of the theory toward simplicity, concreteness, and permanence.

Let's suppose further that such researchers are not content simply to *use* the theory—that is, implement, test, or apply it—but that they are also committed to possessing their own psychological conceptions. This possibility was addressed in Chapter 2, where we noted that a commitment to individuality or to an identity further heightens the effects stemming from control needs. Perspective-taking is affected adversely and the tendency to think in a concrete, oversimplified manner should come to the fore. Accompanying a commitment to owning a unique way of thinking or novel psychological technique is the inherent competition of such a commitment. The consequence is that, if others who are studying the same field are regarded as competitors, their direction of thinking will not be acknowledged.[3]

Let's return briefly to the opening question of this chapter. What happens when a theory is stated in a highly differentiated way, with the use of constructs accompanied by an openness to a multiplicity of operational definitions? Such theories are represented, for instance, in Brehm (1966), Festinger (1954), McClelland (1961), Murray (1938), Rotter (1966), and many others. Our focus is on the *next explainer* who enters the scene and tries to use, test, or alter that theory. There is an overall tendency, when we follow the general direction of development of theories, to reduce sweeping and differentiated psychological statements to zero-variable theories, and if we consider explainers to be people trying to control or lay claim to their *own* theoretical territories, we can see why the direction of development is to the disadvantage of the original theory. The multiplicity of background factors is left aside, and the newcomer, the aspiring explainer, stakes out a territory with the help of a positivistic, "objective," and stable picture of the human.

The control thesis was our starting point and serves as an overall orientation for the emergence of the zero-variable theory. However, when we consider the concrete question, "Why is the further development of a theory invariably in a zero-variable direction?," we see other psychological leads as well.

Superficiality Through Communication

A statement of a psychological theory is one of which the community is unsure. It is abstract, it refers to psychological events that one cannot see or touch, and the hypotheses emanating from it are not yet firmly proven. Therefore, communications about such an entity should follow the same rules as communications about other uncertain entities. It is here that two lines of work have a good deal to say about our problem.

The one direction is that of rumor transmission. Allport and Postman (1947) have observed that passing a less-than-clear story along, in chain form, results in sharpening, leveling, and assimilation of the story. Sharpening means that the outstanding details acquire a greater prominence; leveling refers to the neglect of detail; and assimilation denotes the tendency to rewrite the script in terms of one's own preconceptions. What, then, should happen when a theory is passed along? Roughly the samething. The subtle aspects, meaning the inferred perspectives of the respondents, will tend to be left aside, while certainties (e.g., concrete measuring instruments, external characteristics, fixed behavior patterns) will be communicated in greater detail. The obvious implication is that each successive communication of the theory, in journal or book form or by word of mouth, will result in a progressive neglect of the theoretical constructs, the variables, and the changing perspectives of the human who is being explained. Note that the course of simplifying, during communication, does not necessarily depend on the communicator's control needs. Rather, the mere act of communicating should be sufficient to bring about the sharpening and leveling that, in turn, result in a simplification of the ideas communicated.

Another facet of communication clearly pertinent to our theme comes from Zajonc (1960) and Cohen (1961), and goes by the name "communication sets." Studies by Zajonc and Cohen found that people who communicated about a certain stimulus person tended to transform the background material about that person, material that they had read earlier, so as to remove contradictions and heighten the internal structure of the message. Such transformations were infrequent among subjects who simply read about the stimulus person but did not communicate further. Let's try applying this kind of reasoning to one of the preceding examples.

Wortman and Brehm's (1975) elaboration of learned helplessness theory allowed that threats to a person's control could both increase *and* decrease generalized helplessness effects, depending on certain, theoretically stipulated background factors. The outcome of any given control-threatening situation was regarded as a product of the interworkings of expectation of control, the importance of that control, and the amount of helplessness training. Now, suppose that someone interested in helplessness encounters the Wortman and Brehm statement and tries to communicate it further to an audience or in an article.

It would be hard for this communicator to live with the apparent "contradiction," that control threats could create increments as well as decrements in response. The picture is complex, and an efficient, perhaps more effective, communication of the research problem would eliminate aspects that do not present a clear, internally consistent picture. The result becomes apparent; aspects of the elaborated theory would be neglected in the course of communicating about it. The "contradiction"—that both performance increments *and* decrements can be expected—would be eliminated, and one would try to tighten the internal structure of the communication, as in Cohen (1961). The result is a picture of the human without a dynamic character; a stable, one-sided essence replaces the changeable quality of the person described by Wortman and Brehm (1975).

The Neglect of Base Rate Information

An interesting problem within social psychology has been the observation that the common person, the intuitive scientist, makes a serious mistake when drawing inferences about a large sample or population of people (see Kahneman & Tversky, 1973). For example, intuitive scientist respondents are given the problem of assessing what percentage of the population in a given city is divorced. To assist in making a valid inference, the respondents are given base rate information in the form, "The percentage of marriages that fail in Country X (in which the target city is located) is approximately 40 percent." Then each respondent is given a case history, composed of vivid personality language, regarding a couple just involved in a divorce. It is also noted that the woman had already been divorced twice and the man three times. Subsequently the respondent is asked to make an inference about the percentage of divorced people *in the city* from which the divorced couple comes.

The all-important base rate—40 percent for the entire country—is neglected, and instead, a relatively high rate is inferred, perhaps 60 or 70 percent.

At least two explanations have been offered for this overuse of concrete, individual cases in inferring the characteristics of the whole sample. For one, the concrete case is often vivid, salient, and simply more compelling than dull, lifeless statistical information. Thus, no matter how irrational it may seem to neglect the established fact of a 40 percent divorce rate, the human can be shown to accord inordinate weight to individual, concrete cases, particularly those in which the personal characteristics of the target person are highly graphic (see Fiske & Taylor, 1984; Nisbett & Ross, 1980). On the other hand, it also appears that the intuitive scientist fails to comprehend the relevance of baseline information. Even when both the individual information *and* the base rate information are presented in relatively concrete form, neglect of base rate information is still observed (see Borgida & Brekke, 1981; DiVitto & McArthur, 1978).

Can this well-known variety of failure in human thinking be translated to our present issue—the progressive simplification of theories as they are transmitted across generations?

The Psychologist as Well

The problem that our psychologist-explainer is confronted with is roughly parallel to the inference problems of the base rate paradigms. In the base rate paradigm, the naive scientist's ostensible goal is to arrive at an accurate inference about the population as a whole and avoid a lopsidedness that comes from too much attention to "individuating" information. In the case of the psychologist-explainer, the task is to understand a theory in its original form and be able to test or apply it in that form. This means that all facets of the human that are addressed by the theory must be considered; one's statements about the human are supposed to be structured by the multiplicity of variables offered by the theory.

However, just as in the base rate problems, the psychological scientist commits the error of attending too much to individuating information, to the physically blatant facets of the individual. The concreteness of the individual being studied looms into the foreground, and certain attention-drawing behaviors or highly visible traits come to dominate the psychologist's thinking. At the same time, the relatively pallid, intangible, inaccessible features of the human, information which would be pertinent to a more complete understanding of the person's psychological condition, are shoved aside. Just as in the case of the base rate problem, the psychologist as scientist has trouble making sense of factors that underlie the broader picture of the human. These factors are neglected in favor of concrete, individualized information about the human.

While the base rate problem does not offer us a compelling account of why subtle background information is neglected in analyzing behavior, it does give us a third hypothesis about the collapse of theory over generations. Simply starting with the assumption that the human's attention is drawn to salient, personal, concrete information, or that the human does not know how to react to abstract, intangible background information, we arrive at the thesis that an information slippage will occur as theories are passed along. With each new communication of a theoretical statement, the overriding tendency of the human to attend to the concrete, and not to make sense of abstract, hidden factors, should point toward a lopsided, positivistic conception of human nature.

An Implication: Seizing on the Operationalizations of the Original Theorist

One further implication accompanies the progressive concretization of a psychological construct. It would seem that active consumers of theories, whether they officially do applied or theoretical work, are highly inclined to abide by operationalizations (or perhaps by one operationalization) that were suggested or tried out by the originator of the theoretical idea. Examples are easy to come by. The descendants of Rotter have conservatively hung onto his IE scale as though this operationalization were something God-given, and at most, the extent of the wider development has been to divide the scale into separate, empirically defined segments. Researchers dealing with the authoritarian personality have clung religiously to the original F scale and its relatives (e.g., the E scale), even when an alternative existed (Edwards, 1941) prior to the California F-scale.[4] It is no different in such realms as cognitive dissonance theory (see Berkowitz & Devine, 1989). The early operationalizations tried out by the theorists themselves are the ones that stick; one sees no broadening of the construct in the sense of a wider span of operationalizations.

Empirical Complexity Equated with Conceptual Development

Even if the conceptual structure of a theory collapses as it passes from one hand to the next, it is common in psychology to hear exactly the contrary message: "We have expanded, broadened, refined the theoretical statement." These sorts of refinements are generally of the following sort. For one, the theorist can move toward more categories, as spelled out in Chapter 12. A high versus low public self-consciousness dichotomy is further divided into "body" and "nonbody" public self-consciousness. Or the categories of high and low attributional complexity are subdivided into male and female. Using the geographical designation of the category, one can divide the physical environment into twenty standard situations, and cross those situations with fourteen behavioral tendencies (Champagne; in Pervin, 1981). All of these further complexities are labeled "development," even though they move the analysis toward the Aristotelian tradition.

The Statistical Interaction as "Proof" of the Importance of the Category

Just as with the template-matching approach (Bem & Lord, 1979) or the Pervin (1981) technique, many researchers find that the simultaneous consideration of two categories (e.g., both historical and geographical categories) proves the usefulness or psychological value of the theory. This direction of research frequently takes the form of obtaining statistical interactions between the central category in question and some other category system. That category system can be a historical concept (gender, age, race) as well as a concrete situation, that is, a geographical concept. For example, in work by Heilbrun (1981), subjects were classified according to the S.L. Bem (1974) androgyny scale and also into gender categories. Then a measure of personal defensiveness was taken, as the "outcome" variable. The results showed a strong interaction pattern:

androgynous males showed a low level of defensiveness, compared to non-androgynous males, while the opposite pattern was found among andro-gynous women compared with nonandrogynous women.

"Cultural sanctions" is the concept that Heilbrun uses to account for this interaction finding. It is argued that different qualities of social pressures are brought to bear on women and men and that these pressures have opposite effects, depending on whether the androgynous individual is a woman or a man. That may well be, but in no way can one say that the concept "cultural sanctions" or "social pressure" is part of the Bem androgyny theory. The reason is straightforward enough: Bem's typologies carry no variables, let alone variables related to variations in social con-figurations.

Anderson and Thacker (1985) offer another example. The authors found that high self-monitors received higher ratings in an assessment center pro-cedure than low self-monitors. In other words, the high self-monitors left a more favorable impression. This result was qualified by the male/female factor: the relationship between self-monitoring and making a positive im-pression at an assessment center was found only among women.

Similar to the account given by Heilbrun (1981), Anderson and Thacker (1985) argue that external factors related to social pressures brought about the interaction pattern: "Close attention to situational cues (role prescrip-tions) and accurate impression management. . . should be especially cru-cial, for example, for women moving into upper-level management. . . ." (p. 348). The general idea is that it was presumably more important for women to create and maintain a positive public image. The account might well make sense, since within that context the importance of delivering a favorable image was perhaps much greater for women. However, such variables as socially determined importance are in no way an aspect of self-monitoring theory. A theory without variables remains so, even when statistical interactions are produced by combining the self-monitoring cate-gories with other categories or even psychological factors.

Illustrations such as these bring out a crucial point. Statistical inter-actions involving the categories of a zero-variable theory, *plus* certain ex-ternal factors, are not explainable within the language of the zero-variable theory, by definition. A theory without variables has no equipment for handling effects mediated by tendencies stemming from factors external to the categories. Biological gender, for instance, is neither part of the androgyny concept nor an aspect of the self-monitoring concept. To argue that certain social pressures are associated with gender, and that these in turn affect high and low self-monitors differently is to concoct an explana-tion that is well beyond the reach of the zero-variable concept.

One can produce statistical interactions with a person-category (e.g., androgyny, self-monitoring) in a much simpler manner. The investigator creates a situation (A) that is associated with the behavioral repertoire of the "highs" and another situation (B) that is especially suitable for the behavioral repertoire of the "lows." As a simple hypothetical example, within the context of the distinction between the masculine and feminine types (S.L. Bem), an investigator could confront both types with each of two situations. In one situation (A) the subject is supposed to pick up and cuddle a baby; in the other situation (B) the subject is supposed to try out different rifles and pistols on a firing range. A very strong interaction pattern results; the high masculine subjects show a positive response to the weapon situation but tend not to respond in the baby situation. On the other hand, the high feminine subjects show a good deal of satisfaction with the baby situation, but refuse to take part in the weapons-testing situation.

Does this kind of interaction add particular psychological credence to the zero-variable theory involved? Let's look more carefully at what is done. By definition, the high masculine type tends to show independence, aggression, and self-assertiveness. However, this is possible only if an aggression-furthering situation (e.g., weapons testing) exists for the person. This observation is seemingly trivial. Accordingly, we should not be surprised when the masculine (and aggressive) type shows a positive orientation toward a situation in which one can behave aggressively. The same applies to the feminine category. Bem's feminine person (whose repertoire officially includes empathy, warmth, etc.) could obviously not show these propensities on the rifle range, whereas the baby situation is designed around exactly this warm-affectionate behavioral repertoire.

Research designs similar to the preceding example are seen in Snyder and DeBono (1985) and Cacioppo and Petty (1982); the investigators take the research results (always statistical interactions) to be particularly strong evidence for the predictive power and psychological sense of the "construct" involved. But when we consider more carefully what is done in these paradigms, we see only that a Situation A is created that is especially suited to the behavioral repertoire of Type A, and a corresponding Situation B is created around the usual behavioral repertoire of Type B. One does not need psychological variables to design such procedures nor to interpret them.

Summary

We have examined the question, "Why does theory development move downhill?" and have found three conceptual answers. Whether we look at the longer-range development of learned helplessness theory, Murray's thinking, or Rotter's conceptualization, we see a unidirectional evolution, across generations of research, in the direction of zero-variable thinking. These marked tendencies, generally working against differentiation and psychological thinking, can be examined through the perspectives of (1) commitment, control, and competition; (2) the trivializing effects of communication, and (3) neglecting "base rate" information. Coupled with this generalized trend toward simplification and concretization is the manner in which one tries to build a more complex concept. We have shown that complexity-enhancing efforts take the form of adding categories, subdividing categories, and fitting two category systems together, thereby bringing forth additional empirical complexity. The psychological impetus for such efforts cannot be found within the borders of the zero-variable theory—that is, these efforts at expansion are purely empirical exercises, which do not add anything psychological to the original statement of the theory.

Notes

1. Rotter (1975) criticizes the idea that so-called internals and externals constitute a typology. In emphasizing his point, that there are no absolute psychological differences between people above and below the median on his scale, he notes that the scale mean for college students has risen, from 8 to between 10 and 12, since the inception of the scale. Thus a "high" of 1966 would, by more modern breakdowns, be regarded as a "low." In short, he regards the scale as a possible operationalization of his construct but would not ascribe essences to the members of categories that are created by means of the scale.
2. On the other hand, there may well be reason to think that there is a general decline in conceptual thinking, particularly within Western, technologically oriented societies. This thesis forms the kernel of the next chapter.
3. For example, an experiment by Gollwitzer and Wicklund (1985) demonstrated that individuals who are ego-involved in a performance realm, and whose competence in that realm is not secure, are less able or willing to consider others' perspectives.
4. One notable exception to this monotonic use of the F-scale is a research enterprise of Greenberg, Pyszczynski, Solomon, Rosenblatt, Veeder, Kirkland, and Lyon (in press) and Rosenblatt, Greenberg, Solomon, Pyszczynski, and Lyon (in press). According to their analysis, authoritarian tendencies can be set off by confronting individuals with reminders of their own mortality. The result of such inductions is more extreme ascription to one's own social mores, as well as enhanced punitiveness toward the outgroup.

14
Bringing Psychologists to Study Individual Differences: A Stumbling Block in the Culture

Lest the reader be immediately misled, *individual differences*, as treated by Lewin (1931), must be associated with the Galilean mode of inquiry—with the psychology that treats constructs and variables. Lewin charged that the Aristotelian approach neglected the uniqueness of the individual, reasoning as follows. As soon as all members of a population are divided into categories on the basis of a concrete criterion, each person's essence is reduced to category membership. Individual differences *within* a category of people and differentiations within the individual person, across time and contexts, are eliminated from consideration. The explanation of behavior always refers back to the defining feature of the category—the geographical or historical characteristic that divides the population into highs and lows.

Lewin's study of individual differences refers, then, to the idiosyncrasies of each person. Rather than fit people into one or another static category, the investigator's attention is ideally given to the several factors that converge to bring forth behavior. Given sufficient theoretical background, even highly unusual forms of behavior can and should be accounted for. With this line of thinking one does not formulate principles in terms of "most of the people," "most normal people," or "most Brazilians." Rather, no matter how far an instance of behavior deviates from a socially defined norm, understanding should be possible by comprehending the sum of the forces bearing on the individual.

This sort of analysis should no longer strike the consumer of psychology as unusual. The examples given throughout this book point to such analyses, all of which bring psychological variables into consideration and deal with constructs. No matter whether achievement motivation (Atkinson, 1957), reactance processes (Brehm, 1966), social desirability (Crowne & Marlowe, 1964), self-evaluation maintenance theory (Tesser, 1980, 1986), or social facilitation theory (Zajonc, 1965) is examined, one sees that the theorist's attention is on a constellation of background factors underlying behavior. These constellations render possible the understanding of an unusual, unique display of behavior. Nothing within these frameworks demands that each person abide by the norm (average) of a category.

Some Aspects of Neglecting Individuality

In neglecting individual differences, in Lewin's sense, the Aristotelian explanation does not recognize the following issues.

1. The question of whether people can report correctly on their own behavioral potentials is a problem for psychological theorizing and research. The zero-variable attitude shoves the question aside.
2. The behavioral field that is interesting for the investigator may be subjectively trivial for the respondent. Motivation, interest, and attention with respect to the behavioral field are not heeded within the zero-variable theory.
3. The possibility of the respondent's wanting to leave that behavioral field is never acknowledged. Rather, the zero-variable theory implicitly regards the person as "always there psychologically," ready to exhibit either a high or low tendency chronically.
4. Multiple forces, acting simultaneously on the person, are never acknowledged.
5. The respondent is not granted the psychological liberty of changing from one category to another. The researcher desires that the respondent hold still.
6. The principle that a psychological condition is not always reflected in the same manner is uninteresting to the zero-variable schools. Rather, the manner of reacting *is the essence* of the person, and it remains so.

Our purpose is not to introduce an Aristotelian explanation of Aristotelian explaining by using "Galilean" and "Aristotelian" as explanatory labels. Rather, the reader should take the Galilean possibility literally: certain constellations of factors promote (and inhibit) the explainer's comprehending of the points just listed. Among others, it is a reasonable guess that the nature of the contact between explainer and respondent might have a strong bearing on the final form of the account that one gives.

Perspective-Taking and the Contact Hypothesis

How do we bring the aspiring explainer into the position of recognizing and theorizing about the complexities and flux of the respondent's perspective? The focus early in this book was on the elements that *prevent* such a point of view, particularly the factors of commitment, control, and competition. But what can be done in a positive sense? Can the background of the explainer be arranged in such a way that the complexities of the respondent's perspectives are heeded? Let's glance at a simple idea called the *contact hypothesis*.

High Contact in Exploring Flexibility and Creativity

How does psychological research study the development of creative or flexible thinking in the child? One approach would consist of developing a children's form of the Paulhus and Martin (1988) flexibility questionnaire, dividing the children into high and low categories, and assuming that they have always been and always will be that way. While such approaches are certainly not unheard of (e.g., Scott, 1965), one wonders about the wisdom of studying creativity by dividing people into categories based on questionnaire responses, personal styles, or arbitrary aspects of personal background (see a critique by Mehlhorn & Mehlhorn, 1977). It would seem more to the point that investigators try to get inside the child's world, to discover the nature of their tasks and goals (Getzels & Csikszentmihalyi, 1976), to study the features of their personality make-up that might make a difference in creative functioning (Mehlhorn & Mehlhorn, 1985), and also to find out about the influences surrounding the potentially creative child.

These kinds of efforts entail a good deal of contact between researcher and respondent. In the ideal case the researcher becomes familiar with all of the surroundings of the child that might potentially be relevant to the course of creativity development. Not only can the researcher observe those many environments, but an active attempt at intervention, or experimentation, will create even greater familiarity with the psychological world of the potentially creative child. In experimentation the investigator is forced to pay attention to the hypothetical *future* psychological condition of the person.Under such circumstances it is hard to avoid the multiple perspectives of the respondent.

The Modern Zero-Variable Approach as Antithesis

How does the methodology surrounding zero-variable theory construction compare with the conditions just described?

1. The level of semantics. Instead of an active engagement with the world of the respondent, the zero-variable theorist begins the formulation of the theory with a list of behavioral tendencies that *have* to be consistent with each other, if only because of their semantic qualities (i.e., "creative" and "spontaneous"). The theorist quickly retreats from the actual behaviors of subjects, and certainly from their surroundings and backgrounds, focusing on the semantic qualities of words that are presumed to relate to subjects' behavior.

2. The categorizing stage. Respondents are recruited for the purpose of filling out the categorization instrument, normally in large groups, guaranteeing no direct contact between theorist and subject. It is safe to assume that the theorist seldom even witnesses subjects' filling out the categorization device.

3. Calculating consistency. Without knowing whether or not consistencies on the verbal (scale) level have anything to do with consistencies on a more behavioral level, the theorist takes the answers to questionnaires and calculates test–retest reliabilities and alpha coefficients, to ensure that the built-in semantic consistency is truly there. But again, the theorist has departed quite far from the perspective of the respondents. There is no assurance that these verbal consistencies bear on consistencies among responses on a more overt, behavioral level.[1]

4. "Other forces." How does the investigator find out whether additional factors are acting on the subject, that is, factors not referred to in the central categorizing instrument? Without any semblance of contact with the respondent, these "forces" are assessed per questionnaire, giving us the form of discriminance analysis described in Chapter 7.

5. The behavioral outcome. Even on what is called the "validity" level one sees no evidence of contact between theorist and the subject's world. A common procedure to show the validity of the categorizing instrument consists of asking subjects' acquaintances to rate the subjects, using the categorizing instrument. In some cases the validity exercises go still further toward contact with the respondent, involving actual performance tests or even interactions with others. However, one cannot say that these exercises address the subjects' backgrounds, contexts, or other facets of their perspectives. The experimenter demands little more than a simple performance of the subject, which can then be scored and correlated with the categories.

Crowne (1979) has addressed this kind of problem in his general criticism of the R–R (response–response) research design. He notes that the R–R design lends itself to the *passive experimenter*:

I have so named him because he does so little. The passive experimenter collects correlations between personality measures, or between personality measures and simply obtained behavioral measures. There is no variation of the situation, no use of control procedures. . . . It is all too easy to obtain such correlational data, and the literature is too heavily burdened by them. (p. 225)

Forcing Contact

From the preceding we may draw the implication that zero-variable thinking might well be associated with a mode of research, with the theorist's staying at arm's length from the respondents whose behaviors are to be explained. The zero-variable theory may be regarded as the perpetuation of a stereotype about certain categories of humans. It is both an oversimplification and a denial of the respondent's perspective. When the stereotyping occurs with research on racial prejudice, the recommendation is to bring the prejudiced person into contact with the outgroup so that the complexity of that group's background can be brought to the fore (Allport, 1954). While simply "seeing" or "observing" the outgroup is not guaranteed to reduce the extent of undifferentiated stereotyping (Cook, 1979), it is also clear that relatively intense increased personal contact can bring this reduction about (Stephan, 1987).

Lambert and Klineberg (1967) show that the uniformity, and thus lack of differentiation, of children's views of foreign groups declines with age. A fair assumption is that increments in contact with those groups are associated with age. A characteristic example from the Lambert and Klineberg findings is that among American children whose characterizations of American blacks were assessed, there was a sharp increase in the diversity of descriptions between the ages of six and ten years. The same was found in examining the children's characterizations of Chinese. However, when Russians were the target group, there was no corresponding increase in differentiation, presumably because American children, at least in the 1960s, had practically no personal contact with Russians, nor even media contact that could mediate impressions of Russian individuals.

The contact thesis can also be implemented on a finergrained level. The specific instructions used within empathy and helping research, in the sense of "Try to place yourself in the plight of the other" (e.g., Batson, Duncan, Ackerman, Buckley, & Birch, 1981; Batson, Dyck, Brandt, Batson, Powell, McMaster, & Griffitt, 1988; Batson, O'Quin, Fultz, Vanderplas, & Isen, 1983), frequently meet with success.

In discussing prejudice toward stigmatized groups, such as the handicapped or epileptics, Langer (1989) observes that prejudice is necessarily bound up with categorization. She notes that direct attempts to undo the categorizing tendency are likely to be futile, and that a psychologically more sound approach would consist of bringing the prejudiced person to make *more* distinctions *within* the outgroup, of the following sort:

If we keep in mind the importance of context and the existence of multiple perspectives, we see that the perception of skills and handicaps changes constantly, depending on the situation and the vantage point of the observer. Such awareness prevents us from regarding a handicap as a person's identity. Instead of a "cripple" or a "diabetic" or an "epileptic," we would see a man with a lame leg, a woman with diabetes, or an adolescent with seizures. (p. 154)

One may also bring about contact among two people just by letting them think about each other. In a study by Bierbrauer (1979) subjects made a number of judgments about the behavior of a target person who had played the "teacher" role in a Milgram-type shocking situation. Bierbrauer arranged conditions so that one group of subjects had very little time to contemplate the qualities and situation of the target. Another group was given 30 minutes, but was distracted during that interval, and a third group was given 30 minutes to think and write about the events that had just transpired. Subjects in the latter group showed a singularly high tendency to regard the target person's behavior as controlled by the situation. In other words, a simple interval of time to reflect on one's forthcoming judgments appears to reduce the propensity to categorize another—in this case, another person who has administered shocks. Interestingly, the same pattern of results was found when subjects rated themselves. The more time subjects had to think actively about the setting and the target person, the more they imagined that they themselves would succumb to pressures to deliver high levels of shock. Thus, whether we examine the research on race relations and the contact hypothesis (Stephan, 1987), children's perceptions of foreign people (Lambert and Klineberg, 1967), the direct efforts to induce empathic reactions (Batson et al., 1983, 1988), Langer's (1989) observations on the necessity of pushing the prejudiced person toward the outgroup's differentiated perspective, or the thinking-time factor (Bierbrauer, 1979), the conclusion is straightforward: the "lazy investigator," as depicted by Crowne (1979), should tend to abandon the Aristotelian mode of analysis insofar as there are incentives or pressures toward direct contact with the respondents. The totally detached role of the zero-variable researcher does nothing to spur thinking about the respondent's background perspective; therefore, if we want of talk about a psychology of the background of the zero-variable theory, it would be anchored in the explainer's absence of direct contact with the respondent and in the theorist's reluctance to intervene directly in the respondent's context. One more empirical observation makes this lesson still clearer.

Simplifying the Argument: Contact with One's Own Self

If high familiarity with a respondent boosts the tendency to regard that person in a more differentiated and less stereotyped manner, then we should find especially strong effects when the analysis of *one's own person* is compared with the analysis of another. This is exactly what White and Younger (1988) undertook in a pair of experiments. In their first study subjects were requested to make a written analysis of themselves and another person—a close relative, spouse, or friend. Adding the responses of the eighteen subjects together, White and Younger demonstrated the following: in analyzing the other person, the eighteen subjects employed a total of 114 trait terms, compared with the 64 trait terms applied in analyzing themselves. Thus, our main point is highly evident. Stereotyping, in the sense of implementing categories to characterize a person, is less common when a highly familiar person with whom one has much contact (oneself) is under study.

Corresponding to these effects was subjects' use of more transient states, that is, psychological states, when analyzing themselves. For instance, the reference to specific cognitions was very high (total = 273) in self-analyses, compared to the analysis of a relative, spouse, or friend (total = 71). The same holds for the response group "feelings."

Also to the point is that, in analyses of oneself, semantic contradictions are more frequent. Sande, Goethals, and Radloff (1988) observed that a *higher* total number of traits was ascribed to oneself (compared with the number ascribed to another person), but particularly when the traits came in the form of pairs of opposites. They assume that contextual factors are seen as responsible for which pole of the "trait dimension" will show up in one's own behavior. This kind of flexibility is allowed to a much lesser extent in analyzing others' actions.

Summary

The Sande et al. (1988) contribution underlines further the place of direct contact or experience. Placing these several hypotheses and findings together, we come to the conclusion that close contact with the person being explained results in (1) less stereotyping in general, (2) greater perspective-taking, (3) more attention being given to the context, and (4) greater allowance for dynamics and thus for the person to change categories. In other words, a sharp increase in contact can undo the Aristotelian tendencies in explaining. It is a small step to the conclusion that lack of contact between theorist and respondent underlies the development and perpetuation of the zero-variable theory.

A Cultural Shift: Unwanted Ambiguity and the Elimination of Psychological Constructs

The foregoing constitutes a purely psychological analysis of the explainer. If we take the contact hypothesis seriously, the shift toward zero-variable theorizing should be reversible through the proper kind of training. The explainer needs to become familiar with all that is to be explained, and as long as a minimum of commitment, control, and competition are present, the shift toward Galilean explaining should be noticeable.

On the other hand, this analysis of the psychological aspects overlooks a different manner of approaching the Aristotelian problem. Are cultural–societal forces operating as well? Would these forces function independently of the explainer's control needs and of the explainer's degree of contact with those people who are to be explained? It may well be that the *psychological* preconditions for a Galilean psychology are often present, only to be shrouded or suppressed by cultural conditions or shifts that render the making of a dynamic psychology difficult.

The Pathos of Ambiguity

Levine (1985), in his book *The Flight from Ambiguity*, offers an entirely different perspective from which to view the difficulty in modern societies in grappling with psychological constructs. As a point of contrast he delves into the ways in which "premodern" cultures handle concepts. Some simple illustrations may sound familiar: the Chinese language, by Levine's analysis, is ill-suited for drawing sharp distinctions on the plane of physical reality; an observer gains the impression that Chinese speakers enjoy evoking the multiple meanings associated with a concrete image. The modern social scientist working in a technical environment would react to such language forms with "What exactly do you mean by that?" An even stronger version of the same point is Levine's commentary on the Hindu tradition of ascribing low status to concrete reality (the object world) while the highly abstract idea merits higher status. Similarly, the metaphor, allegory, and associations by resemblance are highly valued in Arabic discourse and in the Somali nation as well. Viewed from the perspective of the current social scientist, working toward empirical precision, such modes of expression would indeed be unsuitable for theoretical formulations.

But let's look closer at the issues involved. At one extreme we can envision a language that has been sufficiently refined by a culture that each term or phrase has exactly one physical referent. When a poet uses the words "black" and "gray," they must pertain to perceivable aspects of objective events and thus depict the color of the night or of a heavy fog. We would not allow the terminology to slip over into the depiction of "gray" or "black" human emotions, to a "black" sense of humor, or to other dimensions that depart from physical reality. Similarly, mixing the languages for the sensory modalities would not be welcomed, which means excluding the use of colors to characterize music or musical terms to describe mood states. The same would be true with constructs in the social sciencies. If a theorist places "insecurity" at the core of a theory, it is necessary to know exactly which physical referents the theorist has in mind.

In contrast with such physicalistic reduction, are premodern and ambiguous modes of discourse simply examples of sloppy thinking that reflect a prescientific inability to deal clearly and systematically with words and phrases? Levine (1985) offers an entirely different view. Ambiguity, aside from the negative connotations it carries in the modern technical world, serves at least two meaningful functions for society:

1. The *expressive function*. An unequivocal, one-operationalization manner of speaking no doubt serves to represent fact, but unfortunately, communication thereby loses "expressive overtones and suggestion allusions" (Levine, 1985, p. 32). Ambiguity in a verbal entity sets off important affective reactions, the arrays of emotions, and also humor. The paradox, the pun, the meaning between the lines, the subtleties that belong to civilized society are all consequences of ambiguity in expressions.
2. The other function that Levine ascribes to ambiguity will indeed bother

the single operationalist. This function is described as ambiguity's "invitation to deal responsibly with issues of great complexity" (p. 17).

Levine by no means offers these suggestions without any underpinnings. A frequently used illustration in his writings is the work of Simmel, who was quite content to deal with dualisms or apparent contradictions within human nature—such oppositions as conformity/individuation, compliance/rebelliousness, or publicity/privacy. These were, for Simmel, the necessary units of analysis, in that man's nature was said to be ambivalent, taking first one form, then another.

Obviously potential ambiguity is involved in referring to one person as both conforming and independent. A rash resolution of the ambiguity would involve the scientist's using some empirical device to figure out, once and for all, if the person is truly and basically more a conformist or an independent type. But here we run up against the perspective of the respondent: the experimental subjects of Sande et al. (1988), in their own self-characterizations, were quite likely to make such ambiguous self-descriptions. If the subjective world of the individual self-observer is itself so ambiguous, it should be the task of the social scientist to meet the challenge and, in Levine's words, be invited "to deal responsibly with issues of great complexity." The alternative is to deny the complexity residing in others' perspectives and to reduce the person, for example, to a clear, empirically defined independent type *or* a conforming type.

Levine (1985) pushes the reasoning a step further, again illustrating through Simmel's philosophy how a sociological analysis can proceed: "Simmel thus conceived social facts to be not concrete, naturally existing entities, but analytic variables, organizational features of human social life to be identified through a process of mental abstraction" (p. 90). Translating his reasoning to psychology is a straightforward task. Psychological facts are not concrete entities, but rather analytic variables, organizational features of psychological life, identified through a process of mental abstraction. Here the reader will recognize Cronbach and Meehl's (1955) notion of a psychological construct—perception, motivation, habit, cognitive inconsistency, and so forth. These abstractions, the inferred psychological conditions, are the real substance of psychology.

Simmel was not without his detractors. For instance, Levine depicts Durkheim as insisting that social facts are no more than a "universe of naturally existing, concrete entities" (Levine, p. 90). Lukes (1972) groups Durkheim with the "imperialistic positivists." One can debate whether or not Durkheim was imperialistic, but the sense of positivism is clear in his work.

It is common that social scientists try to clear the air of seemingly muddy concepts, with multiple referents, by just getting rid of them:

. . . the pathos of ambiguity, a sense that the concept in question is hopelessly multivocal and so one had better fix, once and for all, a univocal meaning for it or else stop using the concept altogether. Such drastic remedies are proposed because the condition of protracted conceptual ambiguity is diagnosed as pathological, for it is said to constitute an insuperable obstacle to clear communication and genuinly cumulative inquiry in the field in question. (Levine, 1985, pp. 15–16)

Ambiguity: A Dirty Word in Psychology?

One of the first objections that a social scientist would raise hinges on the affective overtones of "ambiguity"; it does not sound nice in scientific circles. For cosmetic reasons one could just as well substitute *construct*, *expressions that are not 100 percent reduced to physical reality*, or something of the kind. But let's stay with the ambiguity term for the time being to try out the idea of a nonambiguous psychology.

Suppose that psychology becomes interested in *freedom*. One approach to take, following Brehm (1966), is to of give freedom the status of a construct. Freedom thereby acquired the status of an inner condition of the person, not directly tangible but psychologically *researchable* and *testable* through the variables that were stipulated. Within this theoretical framework the individual's *expectation* of freedom refers to the subjective sense that several actions are possible in a context. The subjective sense of *threat* to that freedom comes about through external constraints placed on that expected freedom. Both expectation and threat to freedom are, with this analysis, regarded as theoretical variables, in that any individual can have more or less of the expectation or threat within a given context. It is up to the ingenuity of the investigator to operationalize these variables, for instance, to understand what contexts set such expectations into gear, and to assess the individual's existing sense of expectation of freedoms. Similarly, the variable *threat-to-freedom* can be operationalized in unlimited ways. These are issues for the investigator to decide.

This manner of formulating a theory is completely in accord with the philosophy of Cronbach and Meehl (1955) and is certainly congruent with a host of other theoretical formulations. But each construct is ambiguous: neither of them is totally reducible to physical reality. And here the Levine issue arises once again—does this ambiguity have a purpose?

The ambiguity of the freedom concept does not reside in the abstract statement of the theory per se. Ambiguity enters when the consumer or researcher has to do something overt with those concepts, for instance, operationalize them. It is at this stage that the consumer tends to recoil, out of distaste for the task of having to operationalize an open concept. One protests that "threat to freedom" means different things to different people, and how is the poor investigator to know whether his concrete operationalization is congruent with those of other investigators? The answer lies in the explainer's readiness and ability to take the respondent's perspective. Viewed through the lens of a psychological theory, the respondent resides in the center of a group of variables: The expectation of free action first must exist or be brought into being, and second, that expectation must be foiled or threatened. This relatively small number of variables defines the perspective of the respondent within a behavioral field, and the task of the investigator is nothing more than coming to terms with the respondent's perspective. For instance, if a certain operationalization is brought into play, will the person's subjective sense of free action be enhanced? Or if another operationalization is introduced (whether through manipulation or measuring instrument), will the person have the subjective experience of threat-to-freedom?

The investigator's flight from ambiguity is understandable, given this state of affairs. Either one works hard to come to terms with the respondent's world in the frame of these variables, or the construct and variables will be rejected. What comes in their place? The lazy researcher of Crowne (1979) would prefer to reduce the construct to something simple and clear. "Freedom," for example, would be translated into the "free type of person." Or "threat to freedom" would be translated into the "threatened type of person," and categorizing devices would immediately be designed to capture the essence of these types. Such an undertaking eliminates the dynamics of freedom, in that the fluxing sense of freedom and threat to freedom are replaced by immovable essences. The perspective of the respondent is eliminated; in its place the consumer of freedom-psychology gains a freedom scale, made up of a list of "free" behaviors. But the nervous investigator has won a few inches of security—ambiguity has been swept aside.

If psychology is willing to allow freedom to exist as a psychological construct, it must also allow that a multitude of antecedents give rise to the person's sense of being free or unfree. The reduction to a "free type" would indeed minimize the ambiguity, but a reduction also makes inferences about the respondent's perspective—to the relevant psychological conditions—unnecessary. And coming to terms with that perspective within the context of the theory's variables is the task of psychology.

Technology, Practicality, and Puritanism

The flight from ambiguity has definite causes in Levine's analysis, factors that belong to the development of specific cultures. In his opinion the combination of the Puritan turning away from mystical concerns and the pressing practical calls of the new world led thinking in North America strongly in the direction of nonambiguity (1985, p. 31). He finds that the flight from ambiguity, and thus from constructs, metaphor, and multiple layers of meanings, is prevalent in all modern, technically oriented societies; North America is simply a particularly good example. This cultural dynamic is reflected not only in the way modern civilization conducts social science, but also in the jargon of everyday communication. Journalism language, for instance, is said to be dominated by flat phrases whose referents are clear and objective. Although Levine makes no reference to the language of modern social science journals, the same element is to be found there, where the tendency to introduce a scientific article with "thing" words rather than through conceptual language has increased markedly in the last 50 years.

Likely aiding and abetting the social forces toward positivistic thinking is a particularly dominant technical element in Western societies—the computer and the thinking style that might well be coupled with its use. In analyzing the psychological consequences of a high cultural dependence on the computer, Roszak (1988) observes that the world of ideas, or theoretical thoughts, is being replaced by the world of orderly facts. A simple example comes from economy, where Roszak refers to an increment in the use of economic "indicators," their complexity and frequency facilitated through the computer. In turn, there is a progressive neglect of the theoretical forces behind economic change. One does not require much imagination to see the pertinence of his example to the zero-variable theory of psychology.

The cultural shift (Levine) may be regarded as a variant of the control thesis that has accompanied us in the foregoing chapters. A highly achievement-oriented society places great value on production and on efficient communication. Each individual must maximize the chances of rising to the top; each person must also maximize the chances of each message being understood, in a manner relevant to planned actions. Given that the achievement-motivated society has its eye on concrete goals, it should be expected that instruments of control and clarity will be favored and the "excess noise" jettisoned.

The Psychology of the Explainer Within a Cultural Context

The idea behind this book is to look into the background perspective of the explainer. There is no practical or theoretical advantage in dividing explainers into Galilean-oriented and Aristotelian-oriented *for the purpose of accounting for their behavior*. Instead, a preferred route is to consider all explainers, whether professional psychologists or so-called naive, everyday explainers, in terms of a viewpoint that should bear on how they settle on and believe explanations. The psychological side of this endeavor has taken the form of looking at the explainer's commitments, at the urge to control, and at the resulting competition among explainers. A budding scientist can develop commitments to a particular portrait of the human, become dependent on that single view to predict and control others' reactions, and, further, begin to strive toward the ideal of holding a unique account of human behavior.

But the cultural context of such commitments and control urges is required to complete the picture. If a society has evolved in the direction of promulgating a language with a positivistic, nonambiguous, anticonceptual character, the would-be Galilean explaining effort is frustrated. It becomes difficult to conceive of constructs—of conditions residing inside the human that have multiple referents. Associated with these constructs are numerous background factors and behavioral outcomes with qualitatively different forms. However, the language that is available in such a technically oriented culture no longer has the power to set off the necessary affects and multiple meanings. It is an inadequate language for capturing the other's perspective, because it refers solely to objective events.

Where Is the Galilean-Oriented Explainer to Be Found?

If the most extreme version of Levine's thesis is correct, then the *non*-zero-variable theory will become a vanishing entity in the modern, technological, achievement-oriented world. In turn, one can look in two directions in search of the account for behavior that turns its attention to the multiple perspectives of the human. The one direction is historical. Assuming that technology and the accompanying distaste for ambiguity and construct have been mounting rapidly, particularly with the computer age (Roszak, 1988), one need only flip back a few decades in the social science journals to find evidence of theoretical statements referring to the broader perspective of the human. Some of this golden age can be found in the earlier half of this century, especially in the works of Allport (1937), Freud (1920), Lewin (1926), Murray (1938), and Tolman (1932), to name only a handful. Shortly after World War II the concept of a psychological construct was made explicit, and a great percentage of the existing theoretical work in psychology was also accomplished in that period (see Hilgard, 1987).

The other direction is cultural. If we take Levine's statement on premodern societies literally, we should expect the *potential* for psychological thinking, with constructs, to be present as long as the particular culture and its semantic systems tolerate abstractions, particularly abstractions applied to the human being.

This does not imply that the most scientifically or technically undeveloped cultures of the world will automatically show maximal potential for psychological thinking and systematic psychological theory. For instance, Lévy-Bruhl (1927) reports certain primitive explanations given for accidents involving man and nature. Among others, a person bitten by a crocodile was assumed to have violated an important tabu and thus to have deserved the punishment (p. 285). Obviously the background perspective of the crocodile victim is not drawn into the total picture. Thus, being "premodern" is not enough. But in the spirit of all the preceding, it would make better sense to answer our question of "Where is the explainer" in terms of factors—some of them cultural—that come to bear on individuals.

1. First, the Galilean explainer should be found more frequently within a culture that is oriented toward the background of human behavior. One element that should foster checking into the background is heterogeneity, surprise, and unusual forms of behavior within a culture. To be sure, psychological theorizing and investigation seem to flourish particularly after disasters that have a human origin, such as war, marked increase in social deviance, and the like.
2. The culture and its use of language must be tolerant of ambiguity, abstractness, and nonconcreteness in concepts that refer to humans. The pressure to reduce person-descriptors to the concretely physical should ideally be absent.
3. Even if the first two circumstances are ideal, the explanations given can rapidly take the zero-variable form when the explainer is under pressure to make commitments to particular explanations, particularly if the commitment involves mining out one's own unique explanation. The social pressures toward offering a better account than anyone else are prevalent in the technological cultures described by Levine; it should be primarily those individuals who are not subjected to such pressures who will arrive at theoretical accounts of behavior that extend beyond the zero-variable cul de sac.

Note

1. In a critical observation regarding many psychologists' preoccupation with the semantic rather than psychological level of consistency, D'Andrade (1965) observes the following:

   The general rationale of the statistical approach to classification in psychology has been the notion that the unity or "reality" of a personality or character trait can be established by demonstrating that some sets of behaviors increase together and decrease together, and thus share a common fate. . . . However, if a number of psychologists are asked to rate the behavior of their subjects, the correlations between items are often taken as evidence for the presence of underlying unities in the psychological processes of the subjects. (pp. 215–216)

   This charge has been pursued since 1965, particularly by Shweder (e.g. Shweder, 1975). But the charge has also been countered—see Block, Weiss, and Thorne (1979) and Borkenau and Ostendorf (1987). The latter authors allow that the illusory correlations to which D'Andrade and Shweder refer can indeed be produced experimentally, but that the D'Andrade and Shweder case is overstated. Borkenau and Ostendorf then demonstrate empirically that personality ratings do correspond to events on the behavioral level provided that the researcher takes into account the meaning overlap among the behavior categories.

References

Abramson, L.Y., Seligman, M.E.P., Teasdale, J.D. (1978). Learned helplessness in humans: Critique and reformulation. *Journal of Abnormal Psychology* 87: 49–74.

Adorno, T.W., Frenkel-Brunswik, E., Levinson, D.J., Sanford, R.N. (1950). *The authoritarian personality*. New York: Harper & Row.

Allen, B.P., Potkay, C.R. (1981). On the arbitrary distinction between states and traits. *Journal of Personality and Social Psychology* 41: 916–928.

Allport, G.W. (1937). *Personality: A psychological interpretation*. New York: Holt.

Allport, G.W. (1954). *The nature of prejudice*. Cambridge, Mass.: Addison-Wesley.

Allport, G.W., Postman, L.J. (1947). *The psychology of rumor*. New York: Holt.

Anastasi, A. (1958). *Differential psychology*. New York: Macmillian.

Anderson, L.R., Thacker, J. (1985). Self-monitoring and sex as related to assessment center ratings and job performance. *Basic and Applied Social Psychology* 6: 345–361.

Aronson, E. (1958). The need for achievement as measured by graphic expression. In J.W. Atkinson (ed.). *Motives in fantasy, action, and society*, pp. 249–265. Princeton, N.J.: Van Nostrand.

Asch, S.E. (1951). Effects of group pressure upon the modification and distortion of judgments. In H. Guetzkow (ed.). *Groups, leadership, and men*. Pittsburgh: Carnegie Press.

Atkinson, J.W. (1957). Motivational determinants of risk-taking behavior. *Psychological Review* 64: 359–372.

Atkinson, J.W. (1964). *An introduction to motivation*. Princeton, N.J.: Van Nostrand.

Atkinson, J.W., Feather, N.T. (1966). *A theory of achievement motivation*. New York: Wiley.

Batson, C.D. (1987). Prosocial motivation: Is it ever truly altruistic? In L. Berkowitz (ed.). *Advances in experimental social psychology*, Vol. 20, pp. 65–122. New York: Academic Press.

Batson, C.D., Duncan, B., Ackerman, P., Buckley, T., Birch, K. (1981). Is empathic emotion a source of altruistic motivation? *Journal of Personality and Social Psychology* 40: 290–302.

Batson, C.D., Dyck, J.L., Brandt, J.R., Batson, J.G., Powell, A.L., McMaster, M.R., Griffitt, C. (1988). Five studies testing two new egocentric alternatives to the empathy–altruism hypothesis. *Journal of Personality and Social Psychology* 55: 52–77.

Batson, C.D., O'Quin, K., Fultz, J., Vanderplas, M., Isen, A. (1983). Self-reported distress and empathy and egoistic versus altruistic motivation for helping. *Journal of Personality and Social Psychology* 45: 706–718.

Bem, D.J. (1965). An experimental analysis of self-persuasion. *Journal of Experimental Social Psychology* 1: 199–218.

Bem, D.J., Allen, A. (1974). On predicting some of the people some of the time: The search for cross-situational consistencies in behavior. *Psychological Review* 81: 506–520.

Bem, D.J., Funder, D.C. (1978). Predicting more of the people more of the time: Assessing the personality of situations. *Psychological Review* 85: 485–501.

Bem, D.J., Lord, C.G. (1979). Template matching: A proposal for probing the ecological validity of experimental settings in social psychology. *Journal of Personality and Social Psychology* 37: 833–846.

Bem, S.L. (1974). The measurement of psychological androgyny. *Journal of Consulting and Clinical Psychology* 42: 155–162.

Bem, S.L. (1975). Sex role adaptability: One consequence of psychological androgyny. *Journal of Personality and Social Psychology* 31: 634–643.

Bem, S.L., Martyna, W., Watson, C. (1976). Sex typing and androgyny: Further explanations of the expressive domain. *Journal of Personality and Social Psychology*, 34: 1016–1023.

Berkowitz, L., Devine, P.G. (in press, 1989). Research traditions, analysis, and synthesis in social psychological theories: The case of dissonance theory. *Personality and Social Psychology Bulletin*.

Berscheid, E., Graziano, W., Monson, T., Dermer, M. (1976). Outcome dependency: Attention, attribution, and attraction. *Journal of Personality and Social Psychology* 34: 978–989.

Bierbrauer, G. (1979). Why did he do it? Attribution of obedience and the phenomenon of dispositional bias. *European Journal of Social Psychology* 9: 67–84.

Block, J. (1977). Advancing the psychology of personality: Paradigmatic shift or improving the quality of research? In D. Magnusson, N.S. Endler (eds.). *Personality at the crossroads: Current issues in interactional psychology*. Hillsdale, N.J.: Erlbaum.

Block, J., Block, J.H. (1981). Studying situational dimensions: A grand perspective and some limited empiricism. In D. Magnusson (ed.). *Toward a psychology of situations: An interactional perspective*, pp. 85–102. Hillsdale, N.J.: Erlbaum.

Block, J., Weiss, D.S., Thorne, A. (1979). How relevant is a semantic similarity interpretation of personality ratings? *Journal of Personality and Social Psychology* 37: 1055–1074.

Borgida, E., Brekke, N. (1981). The base rate fallacy in attribution and prediction. In J.H. Harvey, W. Ickes, R.F. Kidd (eds.). *New directions in attribution research*, Vol. 3, pp. 63–95. Hillsdale, N.J.: Erlbaum.

Borkenau, P., Ostendorf, F. (1987). Retrospective estimates of act frequencies: How accurately do they reflect reality? *Journal of Personality and Social Psychology* 52: 626–638.

Borkenau, P., Ostendorf, F. (1987). Fact and fiction in implicit personality theory. *Journal of Personality* 55: 415–443.

Brehm, J.W., Cohen, A.R. (1962). *Explorations in cognitive dissonance*. New York: Wiley.

Brehm, J.W. (1966). *A theory of psychological reactance*. New York: Academic Press.

Brehm, S.S., Brehm, J.W. (1981). *Psychological reactance: A theory of freedom and control*. New York: Academic Press.

Bridgeman, P.W. (1945). Some general principles of operational analysis. *Psychological Review* 52: 246–249.

Briggs, S.R., Cheek, J.M. (1988). On the nature of self-monitoring: Problems with assessment, problems with validity. *Journal of Personality and Social Psychology* 54: 663–678.

Briggs, S.R., Cheek, J.M., Buss, A.H. (1980). An analysis of the self-monitoring scale. *Journal of Personality and Social Psychology* 38: 679–686.

Brock, T.C. (1968). Implications of commodity theory for value change. In A.G. Greenwald, T.C. Brock, T.M. Ostrom (eds.). *Psychological foundations of attitudes*, pp. 243–275. New York: Academic Press.

Broughton, R. (1984). A prototype strategy for construction of personality scales. *Journal of Personality and Social Psychology* 47: 1334–1346.

Brown, R. (1965). *Social psychology*. New York: The Free Press.

Bruner, J.S., Tagiuri, R. (1954). The perception of people. In G. Lindzey (ed.). *Handbook of social psychology*. Reading, Mass.:Addison-Wesley.

Buss, A.H. (1980). *Self-consciousness and social anxiety*. San Francisco: Freeman.

Buss, D.M. (1985). The temporal stability of acts, trends, and patterns. In C.D. Spielberger, J.N. Butcher (eds.). *Advances in personality assessment*, Vol. 5, pp. 165–196. Hillsdale, N.J.: Erlbaum.

Buss, D.M., Craik, K.H. (1981). The act frequency analysis of interpersonal dispositions: Aloofness, gregariousness, dominance and submissiveness. *Journal of Personality* 49: 175–192.

Cacioppo, J.T., Petty, R.E. (1982). The need for cognition. *Journal of Personality and Social Psychology* 42: 116–131.

Campbell, D., Fiske, D.W. (1959). Convergent and discriminant validation by the multitrait–multimethod matrix. *Psychological Bulletin* 56: 81–105.

Carver, C.S., Scheier, M.F. (1981). *Attention and self-regulation: A control theory approach to human behavior*. New York: Springer.

Cassirer, E. (1910). *Substanzbegriff und Funktionsbegriff*. Darmstadt: Wissenschaftliche Buchgesellschaft.

Cattell, R.B. (1965). *The scientific analysis of personality*. Chicago: Aldine.

Cattell, R.B. (1966). Anxiety and motivation: Theory and crucial experiments. In C.D. Spielberger (ed.). *Anxiety and behavior*. New York: Academic Press.

Chaplin, W.F., John, O.P., Goldberg, L.R. (1988). Conceptions of states and traits: Dimensional attributes with ideals as prototypes. *Journal of Personality and Social Psychology* 54: 541–557.

Cheek, J.M. (1982). Aggregation, moderator variables, and the validity of personality tests: A peer-rating study. *Journal of Personality and Social Psychology* 43: 1254–1269.

Cohen, A.R. (1961). Cognitive tuning as a factor affecting impression formation. *Journal of Personality* 29: 235–245.

Cohen, A.R., Stotland, E., Wolfe, D.M. (1955). An experimental investigation of need for cognition. *Journal of Abnormal and Social Psychology* 51: 291–294.

Cohen, A.R., Terry, H.I., Jones, C.B. (1959). Attitudinal effects of choice in exposure to counterpropaganda. *Journal of Abnormal and Social Psychology* 58: 388–391.

Coie, J.D., Costanzo, P.R. Franhill, D. (1973). Specific transitions in the development of spatial perspective-taking ability. *Developmental Psychology* 9: 167–177.

Coke, J.S., Batson, C.D., McDavis, K. (1978). Empathic mediation of helping: A two-stage model. *Journal of Personality and Social Psychology* 36: 752–766.

Cook, S.W. (1979) Social science and school desegregation: Did we mislead the Supreme Court? *Personality and Social Psychology Bulletin* 5: 420–437.

Cottrell, N.B. (1972). Social facilitation. In C.B. McClintock (ed.). *Experimental social psychology*, pp. 185–236. New York: Holt, Rinehart, & Winston.

Cronbach, L.J., Meehl, P.E. (1955). Construct validity in psychological tests. *Psychological Bulletin* 52: 281–302.

Crowne, D.P. (1979). *The experimental study of personality*. Hillsdale, N.J.: Erlbaum.

Crowne, D.P., Marlowe, D. (1960). A new scale of social desirability independent of psychopathology. *Journal of Consulting Psychology* 24: 349–354.

Crowne, D.P., Marlowe, D. (1964). *The approval motive: Studies in evaluative dependence*. New York: Wiley.

Cunningham, M.R. (1979). Weather, mood, and helping behavior: Quasi experiments with the sunshine samariton. *Journal of Personality and Social Psychology* 37: 1947–1956.

D'Andrade, R.G. (1965). Trait psychology and componential analysis. In E.A. Hammel (ed.). *Formal semantic analysis. Report of a conference sponsored by the Wenner-Gren Foundation for Anthropological Research, Inc.*, Vol. 67, No. 5, Part 2, pp. 215–228. Menasha, Wis.: American Anthropological Association.

Darley, J.M., Batson, C.D. (1973). "From Jerusalem to Jericho": A study of situational and dispositional variables in helping behavior. *Journal of Personality and Social Psychology* 27: 100–108.

Darley, J.M., Latané, B. (1968). Bystander intervention in emergencies: Diffusion of responsibility. *Journal of Personality and Social Psychology* 8: 377–383.

Deutsch, M., Gerard, H.B. (1955). A study of normative and informational social influence upon individual judgments. *Journal of Abnormal and Social Psychology* 51: 629–636.

Deutsch, M., Solomon, L. (1959). Reactions to evaluations by others as influenced by self evaluations. *Sociometry* 22: 93–112.

DiVitto, B., McArthur, L.Z. (1978). Developmental differences in the use of distinctiveness, consensus and consistency information for making causal attributions. *Developmental Psychology* 5: 474–482.

Easterbrook, J.A. (1959). The effect of emotion on cue utilization and the organization of behavior. *Psychological Review* 66: 183–201.

Edwards, A. (1941). Unlabeled fascist attitudes. *Journal of Abnormal and Social Psychology* 36: 579–582.

Eisler, R.M., Skidmore, J.R., Ward, C.H. (1988). Masculine gender-role stress: Predictor of anger, anxiety, and health-risk behaviors. *Journal of Personality Assessment* 52: 133–141.

Entwisle, D.R. (1972). To dispel fantasies about fantasy-based measures of achievement motivation. *Psychological Bulletin* 77: 377–391.

Epstein, S. (1979). The stability of behavior: I. On predicting most of the people much of the time. *Journal of Personality and Social Psychology* 37: 1097–1126.

Eysenck, H.J. (1953). Fragebogen als Meßmittel der Persönlichkeit. *Zeitschrift für experimentelle und angewandte Psychologie* 1: 291–335.

Fazio, R.H., Zanna, M.P. (1978). On the predictive validity of attitudes: The roles of direct experience and confidence. *Journal of Personality* 46: 228–243.

Feffer, M. (1959). The cognitive implications of role-taking behavior. *Journal of Personality* 27: 152–168.

Fenigstein, A. (1979). Self-consciousness, self-attention, and social interaction. *Journal of Personality and Social Psychology* 37: 75–86.

Fenigstein, A., Scheier, M.F., Buss, A.H. (1975). Public and private self-consciousness: Assessment and theory. *Journal of Consulting and Clinical Psychology* 43: 522–527.

Festinger, L. (1954). A theory of social comparison processes. *Human Relations* 7: 117–140.

Festinger, L. (1957). *A theory of cognitive dissonance.* Evanston, Ill.: Row, Peterson.

Festinger, L., Carlsmith, J.M. (1959). Cognitive consequences of forced compliance. *Journal of Abnormal and Social Psychology* 58: 203–210.

Fischhoff, B. (1982). For those condemned to study the past: Heuristics and biases in hindsight. In D. Kahneman, P. Slovic, A. Tversky (eds.). *Judgment under uncertainty: Heuristics and biases*, pp. 335–351. New York: Cambridge University Press.

Fishman, C.G. (1965). Need for approval and the expression of aggression under varying conditions of frustration. *Journal of Personality and Social Psychology* 2: 809–816.

Fiske, D.W. (1974). The limits for the conventional science of personality. *Journal of Personality* 42: 1–11.

Fiske, S.T., Pavelchak, M.A. (1986). Category-based versus piecemeal-based affective responses. In R.M. Sorrentino, E.T. Higgins (eds.). *Handbook of motivation and cognition: Foundations of social behavior*, pp. 167–203. New York: Guilford.

Fiske, S.T., Taylor, S.E. (1984). *Social cognition.* Reading, Mass.: Addison-Wesley.

Flavell, J.H. (1968). *The development of role-taking and communication skills in children.* New York: Wiley.

Fletcher, G.J.O., Danilovics, P., Fernandez, G., Peterson, D., Reeder, G.D. (1986). Attributional complexity: An individual differences measure. *Journal of Personality and Social Psychology* 51: 875–884.

Frenkel-Brunswik, E. (1954). Psychoanalysis and the unity of science. *Proceedings of the American Academy of Arts and Sciences* 80: 271–350.

Freud, S. (1920). *A general introduction to psychoanalysis.* New York: Boni & Liveright.

Frey, D. (1978). Die Theorie der kognitiven Dissonanz. In D. Frey (ed.). *Kognitive Theorien der Sozialpsychologie.* Bern: Huber.

Frey, D., Irle, M. (1972). Some conditions to produce a dissonance and an incen-

142   References

tive effect in a "forced-compliance" situation. *European Journal of Social Psychology* 2: 45–54.

Fromkin, H.L. (1970). Effects of experimentally aroused feelings of undistinctiveness upon valuation of scarce and novel experiences. *Journal of Personality and Social Psychology* 16: 521–529.

Fromkin, H.L. (1972). Feelings of interpersonal undistinctiveness: An unpleasant affective state. *Journal of Experimental Research in Personality* 6: 178–182.

Funder, D.C. (1980). The "trait" of ascribing traits: Individual differences in the tendency to trait ascription. *Journal of Research in Personality* 14: 376–385.

Funder, D.C. (1982). On assessing social psychological theories through the study of individual differences: Template matching and forced compliance. *Journal of Personality and Social Psychology* 43: 100–110.

Funder, D.C., Ozer, D.J. (1983). Behavior as a function of the situation. *Journal of Personality and Social Psychology* 44: 107–112.

Garner, W.R., Hake, H.W., Eriksen, C.W. (1956). Operationism and the concept of perception. *The Psychological Review* 63: 149–159.

Gerard, H.B., Wilhelmy, R.A., Conolley, E.S. (1968). Conformity and group size. *Journal of Personality and Social Psychology* 8: 79–82.

Getzels, J.W., Csikszentmihalyi, M. (1976). *The creative vision.* New York: Wiley.

Gibbons, F.X. (1983). Self-attention and self-report: The "veridicality" hypothesis. *Journal of Personality* 51: 517–542.

Gibbons, F.X. (1990). Self-attention and behavior: A review and theoretical update. In M.P. Zanna (ed.). *Advances in experimental social psychology.* Orlando, Fla: Academic Press.

Gilbert, D.T., Krull, D.S., Pelham, B.W. (1988). Of thoughts unspoken: Social inference and the self-regulation of behavior. *Journal of Personality and Social Psychology* 55: 685–694.

Glass, D.C., Singer, J.E. (1972). *Urban stress.* New York: Academic Press.

Glass, D.C., Wood, J.D. (1969). The control of aggression by self-esteem and dissonance. In P.G. Zimbardo (ed.). *The cognitive control of motivation,* pp. 207–228. Glenview, Ill.: Scott, Foresman & Co.

Goldberg, L.R. (1978). The reliability of reliability: The generality and correlates of intra-individual consistency in response to structured personality inventories. *Applied Psychological Measurement,* 2: 269–291.

Gollwitzer, P.M., Wicklund, R.A. (1985). Self-symbolizing and the neglect of others' perspectives. *Journal of Personality and Social Psychology* 48: 702–715.

Goodenough, F.L. (1949). *Mental testing.* New York: Rinehart.

Gore, P.M., Rotter, J.B. (1963). A personality correlate of social action. *Journal of Personality* 31: 58–64.

Götz-Marchand, B., Götz, J., & Irle, M. (1974). Preference of dissonance reduction modes as a function of their order, familiarity and reversibility. *European Journal of Social Psychology* 4: 201–228.

Greenberg, J., Pyszczynski, T., Solomon, S., Rosenblatt, A., Veeder, M., Kirkland, S., & Lyon, D. (in press). Evidence for terror management theory II: The effects of mortality salience on reactions to those who threaten or bolster the cultural worldview. *Journal of Personality and Social Psychology.*

Hamill, R., Wilson. T.D., Nisbett, R.E. (1980). Insensitivity to sample bias:

Generalizing from atypical cases. *Journal of Personality and Social Psychology* 39: 578–589.

Harré, R., Secord, P.F. (1972). *The explanation of social behavior.* Oxford, England: Basil Blackwell.

Hass, R.G. (1984). Perspective taking and self-awareness: Drawing an E on your forehead. *Journal of Personality and Social Psychology* 46: 788–798.

Hastorf, A.H., Schneider, D.J., Polefka, J. (1972). *Person perception.* Reading, Mass.: Addison-Wesley.

Heckhausen, H., Schmalt, H.-D., Schneider, K. (1985). *Achievement motivation in perspective.* Orlando, Fla.: Academic Press.

Heilbrun, A.B. (1981). Gender differences in the functional linkage between androgyny, social cognition, and competence. *Journal of Personality and Social Psychology* 41: 1106–1118.

Hilgard, E.R. (1987). *Psychology in America: A historical survey.* New York: Harcourt Brace Jovanovich.

Hiroto, D.S., Seligman, M.E.P. (1975). Generality of learned helplessness in man. *Journal of Personality and Social Psychology* 31: 311–327.

Hoffman, M.L. (1977). Moral internalization: Current theory and research. In L. Berkowitz (ed.). *Advances in experimental social psychology*, Vol. 10, pp. 85–133. New York: Academic Press.

Hoffman, P.J., Festinger, L., Lawrence, D.H. (1954). Tendencies toward comparability in competitive bargaining. *Human Relations* 7: 141–159.

Hollos, M., Cowan, P.A. (1973). Social isolation and cognitive development: Logical operations and role-taking abilities in three Norwegian social settings. *Child Development* 44: 630–641.

Hollos, M., Cowan, P.A. (1982). Soziale Isolierung und kognitive Entwicklung: Logische Operationen und Fähigkeiten zur Perspektivenübernahme in drei sozialen Milieus in Norwegen. In D. Geulen (ed.). *Perspektivenübernahme und soziales Handeln*, pp. 429–453. Frankfurt am Main: Suhrkamp.

Holmes, J.G., Strickland, L.H. (1970). Choice freedom and confirmation of incentive expectancy as determinants of attitude change. *Journal of Personality and Social Psychology* 14: 39–45.

Hovland, C.I., Janis, I.L., Kelley, H.H. (1953). *Communication and persuasion.* New Haven, Conn.: Yale.

Infante, D.A., Rancer, A.S. (1982). A conceptualization and measure of argumentativeness. *Journal of Personality Assessment* 46: 72–80.

Jessor, R., Hammond, K.R. (1957). Construct validity and the Taylor anxiety scale. *Psychological Bulletin* 54: 161–170.

Johnson, J.T. (1989). Disposition prevalence and causal strength: The effect of prevalence on the estimated causal importance of conjunctive dispositions. *Journal of Experimental Social Psychology* 25: 36–58.

Jones, E.E. (1964). *Ingratiation.* New York: Appleton-Century-Crofts.

Jones, E.E., Gergen, K.J., Jones, R.G. (1963). Tactics of ingratiation among leaders and subordinates in a status hierarchy. *Psychological Monographs* 77 (No. 566).

Kahneman, D., Tversky, A. (1973). On the psychology of prediction. *Psychological Review* 80: 237–251.

Kamin, L.J. (1974). *The science and politics of IQ.* Potomac, Md.: Erlbaum.

Kelman, H.C. (1958). Compliance, identification, and internalization: Three processes of attitude change. *Journal of Conflict Resolution* 2: 51–60.

Kidd, R.F., Amabile, T.M. (1981). Causal explanations in social interactions: Some dialogues on dialogue. In J.H. Harvey, W. Ickes, R.F. Kidd (eds.). *New directions in attribution research*, Vol. 3, pp. 307–328. Hillsdale, N.J.: Erlbaum.

Kiesler, C.A. (1971). *The psychology of commitment*. New York: Academic Press.

Knowles, E.S. (1988). Item context effects on personality scales: Measuring changes the measure. *Journal of Personality and Social Psychology* 55: 312–320.

Kohlberg, L. (1980). Stages of moral development as a basis for moral education. In B. Munsey (ed.). *Moral development, moral education, and Kohlberg*, pp. 15–98. Birmingham, Alabama: Religious Education Press.

Koller, M., Wicklund, R.A. (1988). Press and task difficulty as determinants of preoccupation with person descriptors. *Journal of Experimental Social Psychology* 24: 256–274.

Kuhn, T.S. (1962). *The structure of scientific revolutions*. Chicago: University of Chicago Press.

Lambert, W.E., Klineberg, O. (1967). *Children's views of foreign peoples*. New York: Appleton-Century-Crofts.

Langer, E.J. (1989). *Mindfulness*. Reading, Mass.: Addison-Wesley.

de Lapouge, G.V. (1896). *Les selections sociales*. Paris.

Latané, B. (1981). The psychology of social impact. *American Psychologist* 36: 343–356.

Leary, T. (1957). *Interpersonal diagnosis of personality*. New York: Ronald Press.

Lefcourt, H.M., Lewis, L., Silverman, I. (1968). Internal versus external control of reinforcement and attention in decision-making tasks. *Journal of Personality* 36: 663–682.

Lennox, R.D., Wolfe, R.N. (1984). Revision of the self-monitoring scale. *Journal of Personality and Social Psychology* 46: 1349–1364.

Levenson, R.W., Gottman, J.M. (1978). Toward the assessment of social competence. *Journal of Consulting and Clinical Psychology* 46: 453–462.

Levine, D.N. (1985). *The flight from ambiguity: Essays in social and cultural theory*. Chicago: University of Chicago Press.

Lévy-Bruhl, L. (1927). *Die geistige Welt der Primitiven*. (Reprinted 1966). Darmstadt: Wissenschaftliche Buchgesellschaft.

Lewin, K. (1926). Vorsatz, Wille und Bedürfnis. *Psychologische Forschung* 7: 330–385.

Lewin, K. (1931). The conflict between Aristotelian and Galileian modes of thought in contemporary psychology. *The Journal of General Psychology* 5: 141–177.

Lewin, K. (1971). Der Übergang von der aristotelischen zur galileischen Denkweise in Biologie und Psychologie. Darmstadt: Wissenschaftliche Buchgesellschaft. (Original work published in *Erkenntnis*, 1, 1930, 421–460).

Linder, D.E., Cooper, J., Jones, E.E. (1967). Decision freedom as a determinant of the role of incentive magnitude in attitude change. *Journal of Personality and Social Psychology* 6: 245–254.

Loevinger, J. (1955). Some principles of personality measurement. *Educational and Psychological Measurement* 15: 3–17.

Loevinger, J. (1957). Objective tests as instruments of psychological theory. *Psychological Reports* 3: 635–694.

Lukes, S. (1972). *Emile Durkheim: His life and work*. New York: Harper and Row.

MacCorquodale, K., Meehl, P.E. (1948). On a distinction between hypothetical constructs and intervening variables. *Psychological Review* 55: 95–107.

Markus, H. (1983). Self-knowledge: An expanded view. *Journal of Personality* 51: 543–565.

Martin, J.G., Westie, F.R. (1959). The tolerant personality. *American Sociological Review* 24: 521–528.

McClelland, D.C., Atkinson, J.W., Clark, R.A., Lowell, E.L. (1953). *The achievement motive*. New York: Appleton-Century-Crofts.

McClelland, D.C. (1961). *The achieving society*. Princeton, N.J.: Van Nostrand.

McClelland, D.C., Clark, R.A., Roby, T.B., Atkinson, J.W. (1949). The projective expression of needs. IV. The effect of the need for achievement on thematic apperception. *Journal of Experimental Psychology* 39: 242–255.

McDougall, W. (1908). *An introduction to social psychology*. London: Methuen.

McFarland, S.G., Sparks, C.M. (1985). Age, education, and the internal consistency of personality scales. *Journal of Personality and Social Psychology* 49: 1692–1702.

Meehl, P.E. (1945). The dynamics of "structured" personality tests. *Journal of Clinical Psychology* 1: 296–303.

Meehl, P.E. (1978). Theoretical risks and tabular asterisks: Sir Karl, Sir Ronald, and the slow progress of soft psychology. *Journal of Consulting and Clinical Psychology* 46: 806–834.

Mehlhorn, G., Mehlhorn, H.-G. (1977). *Zur Kritik der bürgerlichen Kreativitätsforschung*. Berlin: VEB Deutscher Verlag der Wissenschaften.

Mehlhorn, G., Mehlhorn, H.-G. (1985). *Begabung, Schöpfertum, Persönlichkeit*. Berlin: Akademie–Verlag.

Mehrabian, A. (1969). Measures of achieving tendency. *Educational and Psychological Measurement* 29: 445–451.

Miller, D.T. (1976). Ego involvement and attributions for success and failure. *Journal of Personality and Social Psychology* 34: 901–906.

Miller, D.T., Holmes, J.G. (1975). The role of situational restrictiveness on self-fulfilling prophecies: A theoretical and empirical extension of Kelley and Stahelski's triangle hypothesis. *Journal of Personality and Social Psychology* 31: 661–673.

Miller, D.T., Norman, S.A. (1975). Actor-observer differences in perception of effective control. *Journal of Personality and Social Psychology* 31: 503–515.

Miller, D.T., Norman, S.A., Wright, E. (1978). Distortion in person perception as a consequence of need for effective control. *Journal of Personality and Social Psychology* 36: 598–607.

Miller, J.G. (1984). Culture and the development of everyday social explanation. *Journal of Personality and Social Psychology* 46: 961–978.

Miller, L.C., Murphy, R., Buss, A.H. (1981). Consciousness of body: Private and public. *Journal of Personality and Social Psychology* 41: 397–406.

Mills, J. (1965a). Avoidance of dissonant information. *Journal of Personality and Social Psychology* 2: 589–593.

Mills, J. (1965b). Effect of certainty about a decision upon postdecision exposure to consonant and dissonant information. *Journal of Personality and Social Psychology* 2: 749–752.

Mirels, H.L. (1970). Dimensions of internal versus external control. *Journal of Consulting and Clinical Psychology* 34: 226–228.

Moos, R.H. (1968). Situational analysis of a therapeutic community milieu. *Journal of Abnormal Psychology* 73: 49–61.

Mossler, D.G., Marvin, R.S., Greenberg, R.T. (1976). Conceptual perspective taking in 2- to 6-year-old children. *Developmental Psychology* 12: 85–86.

Murray, H.A. (1938). *Explorations in personality*. New York: Oxford University Press.

Nicholls, J.G., Licht, B.G., Pearl, R.A. (1982). Some dangers of using personality questionnaires to study personality. *Psychological Bulletin* 92: 572–580.

Nisbett, R.E. (1980). The trait construct in lay and professional psychology. In L. Festinger (ed.). *Retrospections on social psychology*, pp. 102–122. New York: Oxford.

Nisbett, R.E., Ross, L. (1980). *Human inference: Strategies and shortcomings of social judgment*. Englewood Cliffs, N.J.: Prentice-Hall.

Nisbett, R.E., Wilson, T.D. (1977). Telling more than we can know: Verbal reports on mental processes. *Psychological Review* 84: 231–259.

Nowack, W., Kammer, D. (1987). Self-presentation: Social skills and inconsistency as independent facets of self-monitoring. *European Journal of Personality* 1: 61–77.

Overmier, J.B., Seligman, M.E.P. (1967). Effects of inescapable shock upon subsequent escape and avoidance learning. *Journal of Comparative and Physiological Psychology* 63: 28–33.

Paivio, A., Baldwin, A.L., Berger, S.M. (1961). Measurement of children's sensitivity to audiences. *Child Development* 32: 721–730.

Pallak, M.S., Brock, T.C., Kiesler, C.A. (1967). Dissonance arousal and task performance in an incidental verbal learning paradigm. *Journal of Personality and Social Psychology* 7: 11–20.

Paulhus, D.L., Martin, C.L. (1987). The structure of personality capabilities. *Journal of Personality and Social Psychology* 52: 354–365.

Paulhus, D.L., Martin, C.L. (1988). Functional flexibility. *Journal of Personality and Social Psychology* 55: 88–101.

Pearce, P.L. (1982). *The social psychology of tourist behavior*. Oxford: Pergamon.

Pedhazur, E.J., Tetenbaum, T.J. (1979). Bem sex role inventory: A theoretical and methodological critique. *Journal of Personality and Social Psychology* 37: 996–1016.

Pervin, L.A. (1981). The relation of situations to behavior. In D. Magnusson (ed.). *Toward a psychology of situations: An interactional perspective*, pp. 343–360. Hillsdale, N.J.: Erlbaum.

Peterson, C., Seligman, M.E.P. (1984). Causal explanations as a risk factor for depression: Theory and evidence. *Psychological Review* 91: 347–374.

Peterson, C., Semmel, A., von Baeyer, C., Abramson, L.Y., Metalsky, G.I., Seligman, M.E.P. (1982). The attributional style questionnaire. *Cognitive Therapy and Research* 6: 287–300.

Peterson, C., Villanova, P., Raps, C.S. (1985). Depression and attributions: Factors responsible for inconsistent results in the published literature. *Journal of Abnormal Psychology* 94: 165–168.

Piaget, J. (1924). *Judgment and reasoning in the child* (Reprinted 1966). Totowa, N.J.: Littlefield, Adams.

Piaget, J. (1932). *The moral judgment of the child*. New York: Harcourt, Brace.

Piaget, J., Inhelder, B. (1956). *The child's conception of space* (French, 1947). London: Routledge & Kegan Paul.

Pilkonis, P.A. (1977). Shyness, public and private, and its relationship to other measures of social behavior. *Journal of Personality* 45: 585–595.

Rest, J.R. (1976). New approaches in the assessment of moral judgment. In T. Lickona (ed.). *Moral development and behavior*, pp. 198–220. New York: Holt, Rinehart & Winston.

Rest, J. (1980). Developmental psychology and value education. In B. Munsey (ed.). *Moral development, moral education, and Kohlberg*, pp. 101–129. Birmingham, Alabama: Religious Education Press.

Robinson, J.P., Shaver, P.R. (1969; revision 1973). *Measures of social psychological attitudes*. Ann Arbor, Mich.: Institute for Social Research.

Rokeach, M. (1960). *The open and closed mind*. New York: Basic Books.

Rosch, E. (1978). Principles and categorization. In E. Rosch, B.B. Lloyd (eds.). *Cognition and categorization*. Hillsdale, N.J.: Erlbaum.

Rosenberg, M.J. (1965). When dissonance fails: On eliminating evaluation apprehension from attitude measurement. *Journal of Personality and Social Psychology* 1: 28–42.

Rosenberg, S., Jones, R. (1972). A method for investigating and representing a person's implicit theory of personality: Theodore Dreiser's view of people. *Journal of Personality and Social Psychology* 22: 372–386.

Rosenblatt, A., Greenberg, J., Solomon, S., Pyszczynski, T., Lyon, D. (in press). Evidence for terror management theory I: The effects of mortality salience on reactions to those who violate or uphold cultural values. *Journal of Personality and Social Psychology*.

Roszak, T. (1988). *Der Verlust des Denkens*. Munich: Knaur.

Roth, S., Kubal, L. (1975). Effects of noncontingent reinforcement on tasks of differing importance: Facilitation and learned helplessness. *Journal of Personality and Social Psychology* 32: 680–691.

Rotter, J.B. (1966). Generalized expectancies for internal versus external control of reinforcement. *Psychological Monographs* 1: 1–28.

Rotter, J.B. (1975). Some problems and misconceptions related to the construct of internal versus external control of reinforcement. *Journal of Consulting and Clinical Psychology* 43: 56–67.

Rotter, J.B., Mulry, R.C. (1965). Internal versus external control of reinforcement and decision time. *Journal of Personality and Social Psychology* 2: 598–604.

Sande, G.N., Goethals, G.R., Radloff, C.E. (1988). Perceiving one's own traits and others': The multifaceted self. *Journal of Personality and Social Psychology* 54: 13–20.

Sarason, I.G. (1972). Experimental approaches to test anxiety: Attention and the uses of information. In C.D. Spielberger (ed.). *Anxiety: Current trends in theory and research*, pp. 383–403. New York: Academic Press.

Schachter, S. (1951). Deviation, rejection, and communication. *Journal of Abnormal and Social Psychology* 46: 190–207.

Schachter, S. (1964). The interaction of cognitive and physiological determinants of emotional state. In L. Berkowitz (ed.). *Advances in experimental social psychology*, Vol. 1, pp. 49–80. New York: Academic Press.

Scheier, M.F., Buss, A.H., Buss, D.M. (1978). Self-consciousness, self-report of aggressiveness and aggression. *Journal of Research in Personality* 12: 133–140.

Schneider, D.J. (1976). *Social psychology*. Reading, Mass.: Addison-Wesley.

Scott, W. (1965). *Values and organizations: A study of fraternities and sororities.* Chicago: Rand McNally.

Sherman, S.J. (1970). Effects of choice and incentive on attitude change in a discrepant behavior situation. *Journal of Personality and Social Psychology* 15: 245–252.

Shweder, R.A. (1975). How relevent is an individual difference theory of personality? *Journal of Personality* 43: 455–484.

Shweder, R.A. (1982). Fact and artifact in trait perception: The systematic distortion hypothesis. In B.A. Maher (ed.). *Progress in experimental personality research*, Vol. 2, pp. 65–100. New York: Academic Press.

Snyder, A., Mischel, W., Lott, B. (1960). Value, information, and conformity behavior. *Journal of Personality* 28: 333–342.

Snyder, C.R., Fromkin, H. (1980). *Uniqueness—The human pursuit of difference.* New York: Plenum.

Snyder, M. (1974). Self-monitoring of expressive behavior. *Journal of Personality and Social Psychology* 30: 526–537.

Snyder, M. (1979). Self-monitoring processes. In L. Berkowitz (ed.). *Advances in experimental social psychology*, Vol. 12, pp. 85–128. New York: Academic Press.

Snyder, M. (1982). When believing means doing: Creating links between attitudes and behavior. In M.P. Zanna, E.T. Higgins, C.P. Herman (eds.). *Consistency in social behavior: The Ontario Symposium*, Vol. 2, pp. 105–130. Hillsdale, N.J.: Erlbaum.

Snyder, M. (1987). *Public appearances/private realities.* New York: Freeman.

Snyder, M., DeBono, K.G. (1985). Appeals to image and claims about quality: Understanding the psychology of advertising. *Journal of Personality and Social Psychology* 49: 586–597.

Solomon, M.R. Schopler, J. (1982). Self-consciousness and clothing. *Personality and Social Psychology Bulletin* 8: 508–514.

Sorokin, P.A. (1928). *Contemporary sociological theories.* New York: Harper & Row.

Steiner, I.D. (1954). Ethnocentrism and tolerance of trait "inconsistency." *Journal of Abnormal and Social Psychology* 49: 349–354.

Stephan, W.G. (1987). The contact hypothesis in intergroup relations. In C. Hendrick (ed.). *Group processes and intergroup relations. Review of personality and social psychology*, Vol. 9: 13–40. Beverly Hills, Ca.: Sage.

Stephenson, B., Wicklund, R.A. (1983). Self-directed attention and taking the other's perspective. *Journal of Experimental Social Psychology* 19: 58–77.

Stephenson, B., Wicklund, R.A. (1984). The contagion of self-focus within a dyad. *Journal of Personality and Social Psychology* 46: 163–168.

Sternberg, R.J. (1985). Implicit theories of intelligence, creativity and wisdom. *Journal of Personality and Social Psychology* 49: 607–627.

Strickland, B.R. (1965). The prediction of social action from a dimension of internal–external control. *Journal of Social Psychology* 66: 353–358.

Storms, M.D. (1973). Videotape and the attribution process: Reversing actors' and observers' point of view. *Journal of Personality and Social Psychology* 27: 165–175.

Taylor, J.A. (1953). A personality scale of manifest anxiety. *Journal of Abnormal and Social Psychology* 48: 285–290.

Tesser, A. (1980). Self-esteem maintenance in family dynamics. *Journal of Personality and Social Psychology* 39: 77–91.

Tesser, A. (1986). Some effects of self-evaluation maintenance on cognition and action. In R.M. Sorrentino, E.T. Higgins (eds.). *Handbook of motivation and cognition: Foundations of social behavior*, pp. 435–464. New York: Guilford.

Tolman, E.C. (1932). *Purposive behavior in animals and men.* New York: Appleton-Century.

Underwood, B., Moore, B. (1982). Perspective-taking and altruism. *Psychological Bulletin* 91: 143–173.

Vallacher, R.R. (1977). Public self-awareness and person perception. In D.M. Wegner, R.R. Vallacher. *Implicit psychology*, pp. 85–86. New York: Oxford.

Walster, E., Berscheid, E., Barclay, A.M. (1967). A determinant of preference among modes of dissonance reduction. *Journal of Personality and Social Psychology* 7: 211–216.

Waterman, C.K. (1969). The facilitating and interfering effects of cognitive dissonance on simple and complex paired associates learning tasks. *Journal of Experimental Social Psychology* 5: 31–42.

Weber, D., Koschnik, W.J. (1987). *Lauter schräge typen.* Düsseldorf: Copy.

Wegner, D.M., Vallacher, R.R. (1977). *Implicit psychology: An introduction to social cognition.* New York: Oxford.

White, G. (1980). Conceptual universals in personality description. *American Anthropologist* 82: 759–781.

White, P.A., Younger, D.P. (1988). Differences in the ascription of transient internal states to self and other. *Journal of Experimental Social Psychology* 24: 292–309.

Wicklund, R.A. (1974). *Freedom and reactance.* Potomac, Md.: Erlbaum.

Wicklund, R.A. (1982). Self-focused attention and the validity of self-reports. In M.P. Zanna, E.T. Higgins, C.P. Herman (eds.). *Consistency in social behavior: The Ontario Symposium*, Vol. 2, pp. 149–172. Hillsdale, N.J.: Erlbaum.

Wicklund, R.A. Braun, O.L. (1987). Incompetence and the concern with human categories. *Journal of Personality and Social Psychology* 53: 373–382.

Wicklund, R.A., Brehm, J.W. (1976). *Perspectives on cognitive dissonance.* Hillsdale, N.J.: Erlbaum.

Wicklund, R.A., Gollwitzer, P.M. (1982). *Symbolic self-completion.* Hillsdale, N.J.: Erlbaum.

Wicklund, R.A., Gollwitzer, P.M. (1987). The fallacy of the private-public self-focus distinction. *Journal of Personality* 55: 491–523.

Willerman, L. (1979). *The psychology of individual and group differences.* San Francisco: W.H. Freeman.

Willerman, L., Turner, R.G., Peterson, M. (1976). A comparison of the predictive validity of typical and maximal personality measures. *Journal of Research in Personality* 10: 482–492.

Wine, J. (1971). Test anxiety and direction of attention. *Psychological Bulletin* 76: 92–104.

Winter, D.G., Stewart, A. (1977). Power motive reliability as a function of retest instructions. *Journal of Consulting and Clinical Psychology* 45: 436–440.

Winterbottom, M.R. (1958). The relation of need for achievement to learning experiences in independence and mastery. In J.W. Atkinson (ed.). *Motives in fantasy, action, and society*, pp. 453–478. Princeton, N.J.: Van Nostrand.

Wispé, L. (1986). The distinction between sympathy and empathy: To call forth a concept, a word is needed. *Journal of Personality and Social Psychology* 50: 314–321.

Witkin, H.A., Dyk, R.B., Faterson, H.F., Goodenough, D.R., Karp, S.A. (1962). *Psychological differentiation*. New York: Wiley.

Wolfe, R., Lennox, R., Hudiburg, R. (1983). Self-monitoring and sex as moderator variables in the statistical explanation of self-reported marijuana and alcohol use. *Journal of Personality and Social Psychology* 44: 1069–1074.

Wortman, C.B., Brehm, J.W. (1975). Responses to uncontrollable outcomes: An integration of reactance theory and the learned helplessness model. In L. Berkowitz (Ed.). *Advances in experimental social psychology*, Vol. 8, pp. 277–336. New York: Academic Press.

Zajonc, R.B. (1960). The process of cognitive tuning in communication. *Journal of Abnormal and Social Psychology* 61: 159–167.

Zajonc, R.B. (1965). Social facilitation. *Science* 149: 269–274.

Zanna, M.P., Fazio, R.H. (1982). The attitude-behavior relation: Moving toward a third generation of research. In M.P. Zanna, E.T. Higgins, C.P. Herman (eds.). *Consistency in social behavior: The Ontario Symposium*, Vol. 2, pp. 283–301. Hillsdale, N.J.: Erlbaum.

Index

151